ARTHRITIS TREATMENT

Exciting Modern Breakthroughs

in Rheumatology's Open-ended Future

Ralph J. Argen, M.D. FACP, FACR
(© 2007)

T13 ISBN 978 0-9766599-7-6
 ISBN 0-9766599-7-2
Sts. Jude imPress
St. Louis MO 63112
stjudesimpress.org

First Edition

Printed In the U.S.A.
All rights reserved 2007 by Ralph J. Argen MD

Published in St. Louis MO by
Sts. Jude impress
5537 Waterman Blvd Suite 2W
St. Louis MO 63112
www.stjudesimpress.org

DEDICATION

To my dear helper, my partner, and my wife, Mary Argen, RN

CHAPTER & CONTENTS INDEX

CHAPTER	TITLE	PAGE

THIS IS A PICTORIAL OF A JOINT ABOUT WHICH WE SHALL BE WRITING:

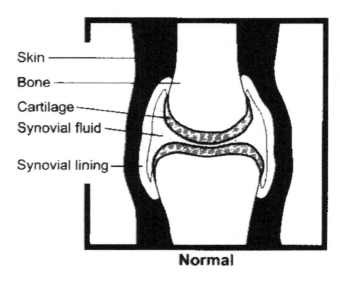

Normal

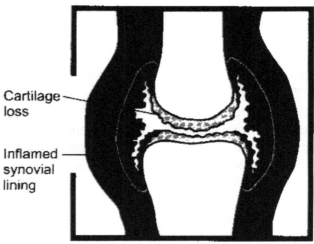

PROLOGUE

In his essay On Liberty, John Stuart Mill wrote,

The peculiar evil of silencing the expression of an opinion is, that it is robbing the human race; posterity as well as the existing generation; those who dissent from the opinion, still more than those who hold it. If the opinion is right, they are deprived of the opportunity of exchanging error for truth, if wrong, they lose, what is almost as great a benefit, the clearer perception and livelier impression of truth, produced by its collision with error".

Put that in the context of arthritis management today and with the new biological drugs and their more or less traditional use is relevant. This and like agents have totally changed and altered the face of the specialty of Rheumatology and the quality of life of people with arthritis and related diseases. Even now fallacious statements are surfacing about these drugs.

Use of new biological drugs to alleviate the pain and inflammation of arthritis has created new vistas of understanding and treatment. Arthritis is now being managed with molecular chemical agents that block this disease at of damage in the joint. The potential of further breakthrough concepts are being extrapolated into many other medical areas of disease. Advances in diagnostic measures, the coming use of cartilage auto-transplants, and research investigation into degenerative arthritis and osteoporosis are vastly expanding the field of rheumatology.

The specialty Rheumatology's future promises that it is creating excitement by these scientific cutting-edge agents that are now available to manage and treat rheumatologic diseases.

Even as we progress in pain relief, many traditional and time-honored medications used by patients with arthritis along with all of the newly introduced drugs are being litigiously and hysterically assailed with two already removed, and others threatened. This manuscript will explain and also defend use of medications long-used and as well as those new to the pharmacological armamentarium for the attack on managing arthritis. This book will clarify and explain the hysteria of today's epoch and offer a proper prospective about Rheumatology; diagnostic management; the proper use of older established drugs; and the status and use of the new agents now available.

In addition it must be mentioned that this manuscript will provide insight into the off label use of these new agents. As a reminder, off label use of treating agents has been the hallmark of managing arthritis diseases.

Data redefining terminology, projections and concepts for the future treatment and approaches in arthritis will be coordinated into this writing.

Ralph J. Argen, M.D.

INTRODUCTION

*T*o illustrate our concern at the beginning of this Arthritis Modern Diagnosis and Management of the Future, we shall show three letters from our author, his comments on recent events are justified and authenticated by over 40 years of practice while managing many thousands of patients with these and all the traditional arthritis drugs. The following are letters written relative to the destructive notoriety that has resulted in denying relief to so many.

The following are three letters recently sent to notable scientists and manufacturers that exemplify some of the concerns that will be enumerated within this monograph - a book that nevertheless aims to give you an idea about the expandingly exciting future of Rheumatology even while praising past clinical efforts, showing why some agents failed, and using the history of Rheumatology to avoid the coming pitfalls that imperil our Industry, needlessly leaving many sufferers in pain.

That having been said, this manuscript is materially devoted to helping the Rheumatoid Arthritis patient to understand his disease, to act in time, know when what where and how to treat his disease and to tell how recent clinical investigations using the new biological drugs are [beginning with Myositis] opening the door to treating other Autoimmune diseases.

■■■

Dr. Gottlieb has been [2003-2007] Resident Fellow American Enterprise Institute: Deputy Commissioner for Medical and Scientific Affairs, FDA, 2005-2007. He was Medical Internist, Stamford Hospital, Senior Adviser to the Administrator, CMS, 2004. In March 2008, he authored an article in Wall Street Journal echoing one of the concerns raised in this book: Congress attempting to forbid doctors from using curative drugs in any off-label configuration ;or for any disease not specified on the label.

Letter to Dr. Gottlieb   March 9, 2007
Dear Dr. Gottleib,
Your recent article in the March 6 WSJ, "Prescription for Trouble" was distressing and terrifying. As a practicing Rheumatologist we truly for

the first time in decades have at our disposal very exciting biological drugs. In this field of medicine for decade's treatment has been trial and error with all variety of agents. I have written two books on the path this area of medicine has traveled.

Recent experience has illustrated the various autoimmune diseases with their end stage names results in precluding them from the use of these drugs. (LE, Scleroderma, Myositis, Vasculitis, Arteritis and twenty others). These new anti-TNF-alpha antibodies block the molecular cytokines and are not concerned with the old names they are given. This kind of medicine is both extremely gratifying and exciting. I am presently concluding a manuscript illustrating most of this topic and the exciting future with these drugs. I personally used these drugs in all the mentioned diseases in a variety of doses with gratifying responses.

My attempt is to teach these names we use are archaic and we undoubtedly have many idiosyncratic expressions of the autoimmune diseases, which need new terminology. I also make the point that dosing ought be specifically customized to the individual patients need and route of administration. Incidentally, I have had extremely good success in injecting very small doses of Enbrel into joints (5 mgm). I was the first to receive this treatment and have successfully and safely used it on nearly 400 joints with remarkable results.

Now to the point, my sharing of this information with the manufacturers who, you already know, will not discuss this with me may boarder on criminality. I would be interested in sharing more information in this area of setting medicine back to the dark ages.
Ralph J. Argen, MD, FACP, FACR

LETTER TO MERCK PHARMACEUTICAL   November 26, 2004
I am a long time practicing rheumatologist and to illustrate my involvement in this area of medicine I have included my medical background. It is my surmise that Merck by its action on the release and withdrawal of Vioxx has been terrible remiss. This statement must be embellished by the assertion that this drug was the best and most effective of all the Cox-2 drugs and added greater safety than all the preceding nonsteroidal drugs.

It is my clinical impression from using a great deal of Vioxx that the fluid retaining characteristic of this and all like drugs is well known and since this is a superiorly effective Cox-2 it's enhanced fluid retention should have been anticipated. Consequently in the presence of patients with hypertension and underlying cardiac disease the addition of further cardiac problems are unquestionable a cardiac risk. This should have been make known with greater clarity. This drug was so effective in instances where indicated that it should be made available again. Only further long-term use will provide evidence of its greater efficacy over other such agents and also its safety.

Merck should again do long term studies of the drug to be used primarily for arthritis in rheumatologists offices for a period of one to two years. Because of the undue notoriety the drug has attained and the legal profession chasing a somewhat erroneous story Vioxx is a good agent is and must not be lost. I would propose the following,

A new clinical trial is instituted with a new presentation of the original chemical.

- The trial could be done over a one to two year study period in Rheumatologists offices for patents with arthritis.
- Reconstitute the drug as a capsule and place in the capsule the same amount of ingredient as a baby aspirin.
- Thousands of people have taken Vioxx while on baby aspirin and the latter is purported to be a heart protector.
- Change the name of the drug, and the presentation, doing as Lilly did years ago with Darvon and Darvon Compound. When problems occurred Lilly added an agent to alter the effect of the original drug and came out with Darvocet-N an extremely good mild pain medication.

The object of the study is to more fully provide information that when used properly Vioxx is as safe as all other Cox-2 agents. In addition since one baby aspirin equivalent is ostensible claimed to be effective in preventing heart attacks and with many patients on Vioxx since its inception have used both, this offers a solution the combination offers justification in these approaches.

There is no reported or claimed pathologic toxic evidence that Vioxx has caused intrinsic damage to heart muscle just as there is no such evidence that one baby aspirin is as effective as widely accepted. The underlying premise in this offered suggestion is valid in such a preparation as I suggest. Lastly the wild atrocious claims of over 100,000 deaths from Vioxx are totally unproven.

Sincerely, [The Author]

LETTER TO THE EDITOR   December 13, 2005

Dear Editor;

The F.D.A. is full of defects in approving and monitoring drugs. It has all the appearance of being too politicized and less interested in drug safety. Proper caution should be provided to physicians and the public, not hidden in the myriad of terrifying potential side-effects in the drug insert and description. When potential problem reports occur to widely prescribed drugs they should properly assess such reports and offer further caution and proceed with the FDA's proper assessment of the claims to protect and comfort the public. What is now occurring is terrible hysteria markedly confusing the public, and it may not be fully valid or necessary.

My clinical impression from using a great deal of Cox-2 drugs is that the fluid retaining characteristic of this and all like drugs is well known. Consequently in the presence of patients with hypertension and underlying cardiac disease the addition of fluid retention can cause further cardiac problems and is unquestionable a cardiac risk. This should have been made known with greater clarity. These drugs are very effective in instances where indicated and should not be unavailable. The action that is being taken is a great disservice to many arthritic patients in need of these drugs who are not at risk from cardiac disease.

The Cox-2 drugs were produced to replace other non-steroidal anti-inflammatory drugs (NSAIDs) such as aspirin, Motrin and a dozen other such drugs. In actual fact these Cox-2 agents were developed because near 16,000 to 20,000 people a year were claimed to die from ulcers and hemorrhage from the use of NSAIDs in treating pain and arthritis before Cox-2's were available.

This activity represents appalling over reaction, with indications that this can lead to more bad science. Another terrible example is claims that Naproxen may be the same risk factor for heart disease. This is complete nonsense. Large numbers of practicing physicians like myself have been using Naproxen in large doses for many years and there is no increased incidence of heart disease in these patients. All these drugs have been the corner stone of maintenance of patients with a variety of arthritic afflictions. Clinically there is no evidence that the incidence of heart disease is enhanced in the patients that take these drugs over long periods and sometimes in large doses. These claims and actions are not well founded with long term assessment of their use.

The FDA, ambulance chasers, and doctors who propagate bad science have done this in the past. We are now ready to add another chapter to the Asbestos sad story, the Silicone breast implant saga.

Promoting these episodes of hysteria do not save lives they add undue concern, frenzy and provide unnecessary pain and suffering to arthritic patients, and unnecessarily destroy industries for the benefit of the greed of the legal system, and fear of the FDA.

People die of heart disease on many drugs and to equate this with the problem Cox-2 drugs NSAIDs and now Aleve is fallacious. One could make similarly ridiculously claims by the percentage of patients who die of heart disease that are on cardiac drugs. The preposterous assumption could be people die taking cholesterol drugs and are at high risk for heart disease on these drugs. One can do this with any drug even baby aspirin since most people who die of heart disease are on baby aspirin. Therefore cholesterol drugs and baby aspirin are risk factors to cause heart disease deaths. As outlandish as this sounds it may be no different than the claim against Aleve, which has been use in large doses for decades in patients with severe arthritis.

This hysteria is the consequence of corporate greed pushing indiscriminate use, hungry legal greed and inappropriate FDA assessment of drugs. There are now more examples of this and they are growing daily. While there is reform of the CIA and national security there should be reform of the F.D.A. and most of the controls against drug companies and physicians are misdirected where there should be strict limitation on advertising these drugs to the general public. This has resulted in over use and excessive exposure.

Patients with arthritis use and have used these drugs and related agents in large doses for many years without the risk and consequence of enhanced heart disease. There is no scientific evidence available these agents are toxic to heart muscle damage or plug arteries of the heart. The mass medial madness is doing the public a great disservice and the F.D.A. is not offering any sense of comfort to the hundreds and thousands who need these drugs for the pain and inflammation of arthritis.

The final preposterous state is the hypocrisy that results in advertising tobacco and alcohol is unlawful, both of which are easily purchased. At the same time drugs that need a prescription by a physician are widely advertised in magazines, newspapers and on television. Since the politicians have lost large amounts of funding from the manufactures of alcohol and tobacco they now rely heavily on contribution from Drug Company PAC's and their lobbyist. Public advertising of drugs that need written prescriptions makes no sense at all. Such marketing should be at very least held to the same standards of advertising as alcohol and tobacco.

CHAPTER 1
RHEUMATOLOGY

> Rheumatology is a specific area in medicine, one that over the last few years seemed to be losing importance but now, in its period of ever-increasing biological/immunological research, pervasive excitement is enveloping our discipline.

*I*nitially, arthritic treatment was primarily aimed at relieving pain with a medicine discovered in 430 BC by the Father of Medicine. On developing more simple pain relief agents, attention turned to treating progressive-debility and deformity. A half-century ago, clinical, or scientific interest was limited to managing treatments of specific types of arthritis. More recently, Rheumatology has become a recognized specialty with the pharmaceutical industry increasingly getting interested causing it to add numerous new electrifying products to its list of popular medications. At the same time, a myriad of non-scientific agents termed 'Alternative Medicine'[3] have also become trendy with many sufferers utilizing them.

A great therapeutic effort is occurring in rheumatology; extensive funding is now becoming directed towards finding agents to treat and manage arthritis. These approaches represent our century's enormous attitudinal change that aimed to solve the blight and pain of arthritis, using Rheumatologists involved in serving other components of their patient's diseases. But the road stated off rocky.

Medical terminology inundates our specialty: descriptive names and terms have frequently added what appear to be separate, isolated diseases to time honored descriptions. Inflammatory Arthritis is a generic term for swelling and inflammation of the synovial tissue and although it fits certain clinical situations, it is not an accepted rheumatological entity. The degree, violence, and various locations where arthritis is involved lead too many non-specific diagnoses, all of which have no differential cause. Some of those varied clinically described entities, such as Rheumatoid Arthritis, Juvenile Rheumatoid Arthritis, Psoriatic arthritis, and many another are primarily clinical manifestations of one root cause. These terms may assist in describing the pathology involved, but they bear no association to etiology. The term Inflammatory Arthritis probably

---

[3] Some refer to most of them as FADS, FAKES, FRAUDS, FOLLIES, FOIBLES, FRIPPERIES, & FALLACIES or QUACKS & QUIXOTEs.

represents the most common form of early, clinical arthritis that exists. Often, it is unrecognized and, for years, it went untreated.

Advances early on in diagnostic modalities and therapeutic agents had been minimal since few pharmaceutical companies in the past were interested in researching arthritis treatment. Although many drug companies existed, each specialized in their own class of drugs. Various companies focused their attention on manufacturing antibiotics, and others manufactured drugs for hypertension and others for other medical conditions. During this early period there were one or two drug companies creating arthritic drugs, making few advances as they went along, demonstrating little interest in developing new product lines. Then, with Rheumatologists gaining visibility, new specific-agents found their way onto production schedules, resulting in an increased recognition that arthritis could be treated. This stimulated greater recognition of very specific rheumatologic treatment programs.

All traditional writings on arthritis state there are many kinds of arthritis and each manuscript adds a greater number of names. At one of the last counts it was stated there are 140 (one hundred and forty) kinds of arthritis. It is one of the missions of this manuscript to challenge this statement and redefine it as probably as little as two or three kinds of arthritis and as many expression as one hundred or more such expressions. The attempt here is not to rehash all the traditional writing on arthritis but to bring forth the state arthritis is in today and the exciting areas that have been uncovered with intense immunological research and its incorporation in to the diagnosis, management and ultimate long term effect and what it will mean in the future.

This area of medicine was originally the diagnosis of end stage disease such as Rheumatoid Arthritis, Lupus, Dermatomyositis, Scleroderma, and many others. It was commonplace in the past to use various agents or procedures to control or have an effect on these diseases. We now have very specific biologically directed agents to attack and control the disease. The problem that arises is these drugs are released with specific designed doses and for specific named diseases. The new era of medicine is not in tune with older traditional ways of designing the drugs and dose to the patient.

The attempt in this manuscript will be to cover some of the elementary ways of approaching these diseases, which are basically, auto immunological inflammatory diseases attacking various organs and tissues. With this approach and thought process an attempt will be made to better define what we are treating and how to incorporate the individualized use and dose of the new agents.

It is no longer relevant to use the old terminology that does not accurately describe the presentation of many to the arthritic diseases. In addition the standard doses of the new and exciting drugs need further design in use and amount.

CHAPTER 2
AN ARTHRITIC EXCURSION THROUGH YOUR ANATOMY

*I*n order to graphically explain the science, the available treatments and the forms that arthritis takes we shall cover the clinical evolution of this disease, increased knowledge, and the agents completely changing rheumatology by touring through the anatomical regions where arthritis strikes, and enumerate their local symptoms.

The most prominent *presenting* features in arthritis are sore, stiff, and or swollen joints. Oft-times, swelling is barely perceptible. Pains during motion and morning stiffness are hallmark symptoms. These may occur in the wrists, - causing the well-known 'Carpal Tunnel Syndrome'- the knees and elbows, or any other joint, or group of joints. For this reason, joint examination is a most important element in establishing the existence of active arthritis. Documenting a patient's history of joint complaints is critical in detecting a characteristic-joint-disease. It's important to determine what areas are involved, i.e., which joints, the amount of swelling, the degree of stiffness, and how long the symptoms have prevailed. These data are important for the examiner to formulate his opinion about the form of arthritis, how severe the arthritis is, and the manner in which it acts. This symptom-and-complaint compilation permits an analysis of the form of arthritis that's afflicting this patient.

A problem confronting treatment of Inflammatory Arthritis and its management, as well as immunologic expressions of these diseases, is that we are trapped with the names of these entities with the clinical findings they are near the end damage they produce. The classical example is Rheumatoid Arthritis: this phrase brings us a picture of a women or man whose appearance bespeaks deformed joint. This liberally used name ignores the early and atypical expression of this disease. We need to fully address such discrepancies.

Arthritis is not diagnosed by laboratory tests. Basic laboratory examinations are helpful for determining if there is anemia, elevated white blood cell counts and erythrocyte sedimentation rate do assist in assessing the state of a condition. Although helpful, these laboratory tests provide information for following the course of the disease during treatment. More important and helpful in assessing arthritis are other basic tests such as

Rheumatoid Factor, antinuclear antibody, as well as additional immunological and basic blood chemistries. However, no laboratory test alone provides data for an absolute diagnosis of Inflammatory Arthritis, or Rheumatoid Arthritis. That is still a clinical diagnosis. Basic blood tests are most meaningful in the following management of all the drugs and treatment used in the management.

X-rays do provide a great deal of information regarding the status of the joint. Soft tissue swelling and demineralization suggest inflammatory disease. The joint space between the bones of the joint where cartilage resides determines the amount and degree of damage in that area. Clinical acumen remains paramount in this area of medicine.

The treatment of all forms of arthritis is tailored to the patient, relating to severity, how it presents itself from the history and findings on examination. There is no specific program or routine that fits every clinical presentation. Treatment is a combination of clinical judgment often admixed with trial and error to find what is clinically appropriate for the condition, as it exists. In diagnosis and treatment, it's important to understand what the patient can tolerate and respond to, and then determine what is least harmful and most effective in controlling that arthritic condition. In present Arthritis Foundation literature, it is claimed there are 100 varieties of arthritis. Giving consideration to the joint anatomy, and how and why it is affected, helps to dispel the common belief about so many forms of arthritis.

Little has changed regarding the cause of Inflammatory Arthritis, or what's now known as hypersensitivity inflammatory states. As in the past, some still consider that an infection might be the underlying element precipitating these states. Infection due to known and unknown viruses or a combination of elements, versus, chemicals, or any combination of these play a part or predispose one to any of the following diseases: diabetes, multiple sclerosis, Crohn's, Guillain-Barré, Tourette's, kidney stones, or Rheumatoid and Inflammatory Arthritis. As a result, major changes are now occurring in diagnosis, management, and treatment of all forms of arthritis, along with reconstructive procedures.

DIAGNOSIS AND ANATOMY

Arthritis is one disease that takes little effort to monitor, primarily because of the sharp endpoint in symptoms, and from input-assistance from its involuntarily involved patient. With patient aid, the effectiveness of various therapeutic agents can be readily evaluated. This process mandates that a prime component of treatment lies in educating the patient about the disease, its form, its likely result, and the desired outcome of the proposed treatment. But today, because of our country's litigious predisposition, most publicity centers on the negatives of an agent or a drug. When a new agent comes forth, its advertisements are initially directed at how it controls the disease, a positive that is heavily counter-balanced by proposing innumerable risk factors turning public attention to how it can hurt, rather than help. Embarking on a treatment plan now presents great difficulty, while aiming to assess the desired result, but potentially bad consequences dominate considerations about any drug that might provide a beneficial outcome for a management strategy.

The basic mechanism in understanding arthritis and its treatment consists in knowing the basic anatomy of a joint. This is the necessary way the medical student learns to understand medical theory; in arthritis, it is our touchstone. The three central anatomical structures are, bone; cartilage; and the synovial tissue that bathe the joint. Although these make up our fundamental anatomy, there are many other support structures includes tendons, ligaments, and a variety of fibrous structures.

Bone, cartilage, and synovial tissue form the anatomy of a joint. A joint has anatomically been described as "the connection subsisting in the skeleton between any of its rigid component parts, whether bones or cartilage." New and rapid advances in the medical management of arthritis by knowing about the anatomy of these components is critical to an elementary understanding of immunology, which today is paramount in rheumatological researches.

BONE

The bone is a dynamic, ever-changing structure following two distinct paths to develop fully. Membranous bone has its origin in the embryo, forming along the margins as cortical and trabecular bone, making up the bulk of bone. The other is endochondral bone, the epiphyseal growth at bone ends: this growth is via preformed cartilage. The primary architecture is a matrix lined with two kinds of bone cells, osteoblast cells, which rapidly add mineral in this matrix, and osteoclast cells that come into action in bone erosion and remodeling. Bone remodeling is a life-long process, which comprises an enlightening, detailed series of mineral transfers and exchanges. Bone may appear to be an inert and static substance, but bone is a dynamic tissue constantly forming and being reabsorbed. Bone's prime inorganic biochemical metabolic elements are calcium and phosphorous.

Its remodeling process involves the following:

- Formation and dissolution of the osteoid matrix (the substance the calcium is deposited on).
- Exchange of calcium and phosphorous in fluid in microcrystalline form
- Incorporation or removal of calcium atoms within the crystal lattice (bone structure is a crystalline structure, and like any crystal can break when weakened).

Metabolically, this process is a simultaneous activity so as to remodel the newly formed bone into a specific structure responding to local mechanical needs; it's an ever-changing lifetime activity.

The bone's basic support structure is subject to many development and metabolic abnormalities, the most common of which is osteoporosis. This particular abnormality, which primarily was considered a gynecological disease, is now treated in rheumatology. Originally, bone structure involvement lay in the orthopedist's domain being deemed in arthritic rheumatology to be a passive substance. It was known that age and Rheumatoid Arthritis cause osteoporosis.

But now we've learned that extravagant cortisone use was also a common cause of osteoporosis. In the past, osteoporosis was an area considered unmanageable, and not easily treated. With greater knowledge of bone metabolism, and from bone studies, osteoporosis has become a significant section of Rheumatology's management of the aged and arthritic.

Misuse and disuse of our bones due to severe arthritis-inhibiting activity, along with reduction in weight bearing contributes to bone loss. This is another modality to be considered in diagnosing and managing arthritis. Osteoporosis is itself a management area we need to cover fully.

A recent plain-X-ray observation, comparing bone integrity of older women living in a northern state to similar observations in a southern state, came to an interesting conclusion: women living in the south showed healthier bones than those in the north. It suggested that the appearance of bone density on plain x-ray evaluation presents a reasonable assessment of osteoporosis - though this at best is subjective. This general appearance, without specific testing for demineralization had simply been considered a result of aging.

This observation was not an isolated indicator but a general one. Conceptualization of this clinical observation led to a nonscientific appraisal of the information. Women living in the south appeared to have healthier bones than women living in the north. A simple conclusion was that women in the north were homebound six months of the year in a state of more sedate activity and little sun exposure. In the south, women had greater outdoor physical activity with sun-exposure resulting in an increase in vitamin D entering the body, hence healthier bones. This purely non-scientific deduction needs a scientific demographic population study. A study of the incidence of various hip, wrist and spinal compression fractures, factored into age in northern or southern localities might add credence to this suggestion.

CARTILAGE

Articular cartilage is a tough, resilient connective tissue comprised of cells and fibers embedded in a firm, gel-like matrix. It contains chondroitin sulfate, A and C. Adult cartilage has neither nerves nor blood vessels within it. Articular cartilage has an elastic characteristic not visualized. When compressed, it gets thinner but, when pressure is released, it regains its original thickness. Intermittent pressure on cartilage appears to cause it to take up fluid, giving it a sponge-like character. This allows it to absorb synovial fluid from which it receives nourishment. Cartilage-surface is comprised of undulating tightly-woven fiber bundles, which, in turn, have micro-convolutions that contribute roughness to a normal surface. In short, articular cartilage resembles a stiff sponge having elastic character. It is able to absorb fluid, and capable of exuding fluid: an important mechanism in lubricating the joint. Cartilage anatomy, in its description and function, is a dynamic structure, not the inert substance it is frequently considered to be. On taking into account the dynamic character of cartilage, the difficulty of altering it surgically becomes understandable.

Disease of this substance represents a specific form of arthritis. Cartilage supposedly can be damaged by wear and tear or trauma, resulting in pain and ultimately in joint dysfunction. This results in what is called osteoarthritis. Even having just enumerated cartilage as a tough, resilient connective tissue composed of cells and fibers embedded in a firm, gel-like matrix, greater knowledge and interest in cartilage has resulted and will result in naturally enhancing and replacing cartilage with natural substances.

One result is the common use of a recent, over the counter agent called chondroitin sulfate. Orally, it is used as a natural component for the treatment of arthritis. Yet, this has little scientific efficacy. As mentioned, articular cartilage receives much of its nourishment from the synovial fluid. A healthy synovium produces healthy cartilage; an ailing synovium enhances damage to articular cartilage.

During normal activity, articular cartilage remains healthy in spite of being subjected to massive forces. Articular cartilage is extremely resilient, withstanding enormous pounds per square inch [p.s.i.], with compression, gliding, and searing forces during normal use. With abnormal physical use and heavy weight bearing, cartilage is subject to damage. Joints architecturally are master-engineered to sustain massive forces, which occur during all manner of use.

One active protective mechanism is muscle contraction support. Three more passive protective mechanisms are:

- Transference of forces to surrounding tissue, the soft tissue, and ligaments as the joint load increases. The joint is then able to allow greater contact to a larger surface and support an effectively increased joint area;
- Compliance of cartilage and callous bone also has a protective mechanism;
- Bone ends are flared, offering a greater surface to bear force.

An important negative about articular cartilage is that it has poor capability for self-repair. Were enhancement of cartilage repair to become available in the future, cartilage transplants might be used to treat arthritis and joint disease.

Transplantation of autologus cartilage has been cultivated and utilized, but whether it will be effective over time is yet to be determined. The property of articular cartilage, as with all tissue, is that its biochemical and structural characteristics alter with age. These changes result in decreased stiffness to the cartilage, causing it to be subject to injury with a potential for developing osteoarthritis, the cartilage disease.

SYNOVIAL MEMBRANE

The synovial membrane is a vascular connective tissue lining the inner surface of joint cavities. It does not cover the articular cartilage. Visually, it's a glossy substance with a relatively smooth surface out of which exudes a variety of villi and fat pads that project into the joint space. This highly vascular tissue can reproduce, and provide nourishment for the joint; it's the structure primarily responsible for arthritic debilitation.

Synovial tissue is the anatomical component behind destruction in inflammatory joint disease. The synovial membrane is the structure within the joint, whose abnormal proliferation is the prime cause of the destructive damage to cartilage in Rheumatoid Arthritis, when it becomes inflamed. When injurious changes occur, erosive damage inflicts the cartilage, with injury to cortical bone. Years later, it was determined that synovial tissue provides very harmful material, causing local harm to articular cartilage. All treatment for inflammatory joint disease is specifically directed at the synovial tissue.

These three anatomical subsets are appraised in diagnosing, treating, and managing every form of arthritis. Originally, this almost imperceptible synovial tissue, isn't easily seen, felt, or examined, so it was given only modest consideration in coming to grips with joint disease dynamics.

In early literature, the synovium may have been conceptualized but it was rarely awarded clinical perception nor was it actually examined. As the caseload of joint surgery increased, and with the use of joint aspiration and injection, closer attention was given to the synovium. The joint fluid acquired by aspiration when inspected, became a target of interest and general testing. Many a researcher hoped that, via microscopic examination of the synovial fluid, they could better determine disease severity and specificity.

Synovial lining cells lie loosely in a bed of hylauronate interspersed with collagen. This macromolecular sieve is what gives the tissue its semi-permeable characteristic. As stated before, the synovium nourishes and produces the synovial fluid that bathes the joints. This abundantly vascular tissue, when being well evaluated, provided no clue to the specific character of the diseased tissue. Microscopic examination of synovial tissue did not, and will not, reveal its form of joint disease, or predict its coming degree of severity.

Synovial biopsy was once considered important for providing precise diagnostic information about arthritis. The synovium, when diseased, can act only in a minimal number of ways regardless of its inciting agency: A debilitated synovium becomes swollen, edematous, vascular, and locally destructive. No happy clue resides in this tissue to provide a specific diagnosis.

When the disease is long-standing, or when metabolic abnormalities abound as in severe Rheumatoid Arthritis, or gout, specific findings exist: research has determined whether examination of the fluid might reveal information as to the severity and cause of Inflammatory Arthritis. As in most tests, it is a helpful agent but doesn't provide definitive or actual diagnostic information. Synovial tissue evaluation is quite helpful though it's not as specific as joint aspiration in gout or infectious arthritis, which can be exact.

Advances in reconstructive surgery have allowed us to actually see and further experience live, actively destructive synovial tissue. When synovium becomes swollen and markedly proliferate, it's so locally destructive that one could almost make a case for it acting as a local malignancy, which it is not. This is the tissue where therapeutic attention is directed for inflammatory joint disease, to decrease its proliferation, and minimize swelling, or arrest the damage it is producing. Over the years, essential knowledge has resulted by studying this tissue. Even so, we still have great difficulty in altering its activity, and the effect it has on basic joint structure.

For years, treating this synovial inflammation and the destruction it causes to cartilage seemed hopeless. At this time, there's evidence suggesting that we can now alter this damaging process. Further delving into the biochemical immunologic findings now allow clinicians to more fully understand, manage and treat inflamed synovial tissue causing basic joint damage.

SYNOVIAL FLUID

This joint lubricating fluid is central to joint activity. Knowledge of the synovial fluid can inform us about what's occurring in the joint itself. Contrary to what's been stated, the synovial tissue itself is not definitively specific, nor can an examiner easily access it. Synovial fluid is just the opposite: needle aspiration is a snap to perform, and can be quite revealing. Its basic appearance during aspiration tells a great deal concerning just what is occurring in the joint. Normally, the quantity of synovial fluid, which is essential for lubrication and nutrition, is no more than half a teaspoon [~2.5 ml]. If any cells are present in the synovial fluid, they are minimal, and this yellowish fluid is usually clear. It is quite viscous and, when poured, has a stringy character. An increase in the quantity of fluid may result from a variety of reasons, depending on the joint pathology.

Simple traumatic wear-and-tear is usually associated with an increased fluid of relative normal character. In more acute trauma, blood can easily be discerned. In an inflamed arthritic joint, the fluid is cloudy, less viscous, all of which can be seen with a brief inspection during initial aspiration. An infected joint has a great number of white cells and bacteria all of which, again, are easily detected. In metabolic problems, there are occasions as with gout, crystals are found in the joint. This adds to the underlying pathology, and is the causative factor in gouty arthritis. Microscopic examination of joint fluid provides further information, and occasionally, the fluid may warrant culturing for bacteria and infection.

COLLAGEN

Collagen is another tissue composing part of the arthritis structure. It is loosely defined as a supporting or connective tissue. Before there was much specificity regarding this tissue, diseases of this basic support tissue were defined as connective tissue disorders, or collagen diseases. Collagen and elastin are both composed of fibrous proteins, but they are different. Collagen is a highly ordered assembly having a microbiological structure; elastin does not. We have identified at least nineteen different types of collagen. Collagen is connective tissue's least common denominator in disease structure. This basic tissue is bio-chemical and genetic; it has found a world of its own. Although where rheumatic diseases are involved, the information on collagen gathered in the last few decades has had little impact on diseases management or treatment. Its long-term effect on further biochemical knowledge will result in greater specificity in our pharmacological approach to treatment. Although cures lay distant, newer agents are helping us to move closer. Collagen's basic structure must be more fully understood to better understand the mechanism creating primary inflammation of any and all tissue.

THE SPINE

The spine is an entire organ unto itself with respect to arthritis. Anything that involves the peripheral joints, such as inflammation, strain, degeneration, and trauma will involve the spine as well. The spine consists of seven cervical, twelve thoracic, and five lumbar vertebrae – all being jointed together. Between each vertebra are discs, which act to absorb shock. Note also that these structures are protecting the spinal cord in which nerve roots originate.

Concerning the spine, considerable attention needs be given to its musculoskeletal system because of its complex structure and the wide variety of problems that may occur. These include Inflammatory Arthritis known as Ankylosing Spondylitis, degenerative joint disease, disc disease, as well as pathology in the bone itself. Each segment of the spine bears its own set of problems and symptoms. Because of all the structures and nerve roots involved, the findings and diagnoses can be complex. There are a wide variety of therapeutic approaches to diseases of the spine, but the critical element is a high index of suspicion, critical evaluation, and conservative management.

In these problems, there is an extensive diversity of accepted modalities, but because of the complexity of the problems and diagnoses, an even larger number of non-scientific methods are frequently attempted. One cannot give enough stress to the patient that: 'a conservative approach is the most reasonable and effective route to follow'. There are no easy cures or shortcuts to manage and treat symptoms and diseases of the spine.

CHAPTER 3

CELLULAR AND BIOLOGICAL PATHOLOGY OF JOINT DISEASE

Modern rheumatology has advanced in understanding the pathology that's occurring in a diseased joint. Along with this knowledge, specific biological immunological management and treatment is developing. This has added an entirely new perception towards understanding the pathological process in arthritis.

The cellular and anatomic location and structure of the joint has been described but, primarily or secondarily, it is in the synovium where disease activity is actually highlighted. What is being alluded to in that statement is that the synovium is the primary scene of disease's attack? Synovium tissue perpetuates the damage or causes the secondary damage to cartilage; inflammatory activity then provokes further damage. In this chapter we will attempt to define out body's molecular players lying behind our immune system's attack on its own tissues. But before embarking upon this complex topic, a word about what is precipitating this discussion on autoimmunity.

RA IS AN AUTOIMMUNE DISEASE

This medical book desires to present matters not written about in most standard texts and monographs. It's aimed at the larger number of patients with RA, a disease that can completely remit - sometimes never only to return, or return many years later wearing a different expression.

RA is considered an autoimmune disease in which the immune system is producing immune factors attacking ones own synovial tissue. Genetic factors may play a role in why this occurs in some individuals. The presence of an antibody in a significant number of RA patients with rheumatic Inflammatory Arthritis lends support to some degree of a genetic predisposition towards acquiring this disease. Rheumatoid Factor (RF), the antibody to an immune substance (IgG), was one of the early blood serum elements that was considered its disease marker. Often and again, this has been searched for in tests to establish the diagnosis of RA. It may be present in 70% of cases. Most people waiting for these diagnostic blood serological tests will suffer for years undiagnosed while wasting elsewhere-needed money, as well as years before their correct treatment commences. Too much attention has been paid to this specific antibody test, not for diagnosing the patient, just to help in finding the origin of RA.

High titers of RF written about are considered associated with more severe and active joint disease, having greater systemic involvement, and a poorer prognosis for remission. RA, as well as other autoimmune diseases, includes widespread immunologic and inflammatory alterations of connective tissue. Because the so-called autoimmune diseases share many clinical-findings, a differential diagnosis is often made difficult. Although the autoimmune disorders are considered acquired diseases, their causes usually cannot be determined. Systemic serological findings being too frequently relied upon don't correlate with the clinical picture. That's why these tests frighten individuals by what they have read on-line, or in books.

The cellular and immunological data and elements in this important tissue are briefly surveyed, described, and listed below.

OUR BODY'S IMMUNE AND AUTOIMMUNE SYSTEM

The immune system is a Surveillance Patrol. Its uncountable patrolmen flow from the Thymus, and Bone Marrow through the blood and lymph streams looking for culprits that have invaded the body. They identify them as not being homebodies and destroy them. These interlopes include bacteria, viruses, microbes, proto-cancer cells and fungi coming from cuts to the skin, or from breathing and swallowing. These are recognized as antigens [things that are not genetically me]. It's an almost miraculous system since; if it did not exist, no baby would survive her first swig of non-mother-milk, or his first gulp of water, or first deep breath. (If that seems unlikely consider histories of babies forever encased in a bacteria-free balloon.)

But sometimes, the well-trained patrol identifies something in the body as an outsider and calls on its antibody squads to wipe it out. The immune system memorizes the molecules on its new enemy and places that identification on new stem cell patrolmen that reproduce themselves as needed. Those squads are trained to find and kill. These killers are called 'Autoantibodies' and, in every drop of blood, there are thousands of them with orders to kill the enemy one at a time [since there are multimillions of such enemies. For many autoimmune diseases, the autoimmune cells that are flowing do not complete their destruction quickly, as arthritis sufferers can testify.

It's been by developing biological cells that attack the attacks that Rheumatology is on its way to a solution, but that path has such an uncommon language that a reader needs to learn its words and terms. So here's our primer on the Immune System [skip it if you wish but know that it will still be here]:

YOUR IMMUNE SYSTEM

The Immune system can be divided into two parts: the first is the natural system whose patrols inherently recognize cells known to be not part of the body. To recognize an enemy, the body adds receptor sites onto the patrolmen.

Not all invaders are innately recognized from birth since viruses do mutate into new forms. The second part of the system acquires specific knowledge how an invader is not "I". Adaptive immunity specifically develops protective substances after being exposed to new attackers getting through its protecting organs: skin, mucous, and lung lining.

FIRST IS NATURAL (innate) IMMUNITY

The system has three kinds of Interferons whose purpose is to inhibit an intruder from replicating itself. Interferons are made from/by cells that have been infected by this intruding antigen. Interferons fall into three types:

- Interferon-α [from non-Lymphocyte white blood cells];
- Interferon-β [from Fibroblasts];
- Interferon-γ [from Lymphocytes].

Then, there are Scavenger cells called Microphages and Macrophages; both are able to ingest intruders:

* Microphages (little eaters filled with digestive enzymes) [a.k.a Granulocyte-Leukocytes] are manufactured from stem cells produced by the bone marrow. There are three types: Neutrophils; Eosophils and Basophils Neutrophils are so predominant that they are considered the microphage.

* Macrophages (big eaters) are derived from Monocytes, which also come from stem cells under continuous fabrication, by the Thymus Gland and Bone Marrow. Its flock of enzymes gobble up intruders, and then the macrophage sends out signals causing battalions of leukocytes [white blood cells] to join the fray.

The third group is termed NK [natural killers]. These are fabricated from lymphocyte granulocytes that are stimulated by -Interferon. Further protection comes with the body raising a fever. This is termed the ACUTE PHASE in which proteins form from the liver and Interleukin (IL-1).

This diagram may assist while perusing the upcoming paragraphs.

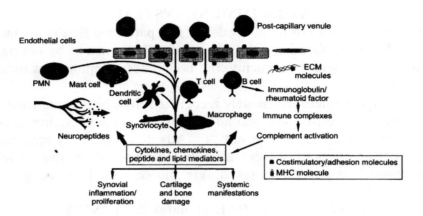

THEN THERE'S OUR ADAPTIVE, i.e. specific IMMUNITY

Of the two trillion [bone marrow formed] lymphocytes in the body, twenty million flow through the blood stream. They flow into the Thymus Gland and into the Bone Marrow. Inside them, these white cells get attached with receptors sites that complement molecule sites found on at least a quarter of a million different kinds of foreigners. They then flow through the blood and the lymph streams looking for matches they can bind onto and kill while, at the same time, replicating themselves to find every other such intruder. Some of the molecules pertinent to RA include:

CD45TRO
CD29bright
CD11a/CD18(LFA-1)
VLA-1
CD49d/CD29
CD54
CD44
CD7dim

Cells coming out of the Thymus are called T-cells, and those exiting the marrow are B-cells.

B-cells secrete antibodies [immunoglobins] with receptors that complement the antigens. These antibodies flow through the lymph-stream.

T-cells do the killing job themselves while multiplying [via polyclonal mutagenesis]. There are two types of T-cells: Helpers and Cytotoxins [Suppressors].

T cells send signals to messenger molecules called cytokines.

Cytokines can activate immune cells. One of the cytokines that cause inflammation is called TNF-α (*tumor necrosis factor alpha*).

Cytokines act like magnets for other immune cells. Over production of cytokines attracts macrophages and other destructive cells called Neutrophils - also called Stagocytes. They destroy invaders with toxic molecules sending out signals to T cells sometimes sending out too many giving rise to an autoimmune response to destroy cells in nerves and joints. Cytokines have demonstrated the ability to damage articular cartilage and bone. Some such proven substances are:

IL-1

TNF-α

TNF-g

IL-6

Now the problem with our adaptive autoimmune system is that, for a completely unknown reason, it mysteriously and mistakenly discovers that some of a person's good cells are bad guys, and so antibodies and cytokines are sent out to destroy them. There are at least thirty autoimmune diseases but, in this manuscript, we are focusing in on just one of them: Arthritis [and the synovium].

THE SYNOVIUM.

It is just one to three cell layers thick. These synovial cells are Synoviocytes of Type A: Macrophage; and Type B: Fibroblast [leukocyte]

During inflammation, the synovium increases as it proliferates, causing swelling and from blood vessel engorgement called angiogenesis.

Its sequence involves:

- Infiltration of inflammatory cells
- Chemotactic stimulation;
- Introduction of proinflammatory cytokines;
- T lymphocytes, and
- B lymphocytes, and
- Increased leukocytes, and
- Mononuclear cells;
- Monoplanes, and
- Plasma cells;

- CD4+ helper T cells,
- Antigen presenting cells
- Macrophages;
- Dendrite cells.

Cellular activity in the synovium's three layers includes:

Memory T cells;

Helper B cells; and

Immunoglobulin synthesis.

- Lymphocytes form Lymphoid Follicles;
- In the transitional region, Lymphocyte Blasts and Lymphocytes lying in close proximity to HLA-A-DR+ (an activating antigen);
- This plasma rich area is responsible for immunoglobulin and RF.

One can presume all these ARTHRIDITIES in the synovium, and all these described immunological and biological chemicals, antibodies and molecules, will act the same regardless of the name we have given the disease involved. This statement promotes impact to the earlier comment that <u>arthritis may be just a primary disease of synovial tissue</u> or secondary mechanical damage to articular cartilage causing secondary synovial inflammation producing the same synovial changes. Therefore, if each form differs only in the amount of attackers, there may be only one or two actual forms of arthritis with over one hundred different expressions in form and magnitude.

The following groups of synovial attackers denote present day findings about synovial inflammation activity occurring in arthritis, and how we are now assessing the disease and its management.

- Cytokines [These are proteins acting as mediators];
- TNF-α [Tumor Necrosis Factor];
- Interleukins IL-3, IL-4;
- TGF-β (Transforming Growth Factor).

The underlying cause for all this proliferation and inflammatory immunological activity in the synovium is open yet too everyone's speculation. This is most likely an antigen producing disease that sets off the immune system.

Cells contribute to the inflammatory process by secreting vasoactive material. Also open to confirmed speculation are the rolls of various cells such as: Circulating memory cells; Tissue macrophages; Cytokines and Plasma cells in the process.

As for specific cytokines many have already been identified -from T-cell research discoveries over the last few years - among them are:

IL-1
TNF-α
IFN-g (interferon- gamma)
TGF-β
IL-8
Causing activation of many cell types to name a few
IL-1
IL-2
IFN-g
TNF-
IL-6
IL-10
GM-CSF

Clinical features cannot be collectively categorized as to the kind of synovial damaging activity, which is associated with any named arthritis disease. Each arthritic disease owns its unique clinical expressions. Knowing more about its immuno-pathology, it is counter productive to attach colorful names to various expressions of synovial inflammatory disease. In the future genetic typing may offer more to attaching names and prognosis.

In summation there are numerous cells and cellular interactivity and cellular substances involved in the inflammatory, proliferative and damaging activities in and from the synovium.

FIGHTING THE CYTOKINES:
The modern era of management and understanding synovial disease began with the use of the first new biological agent, details about these will be presented in a later chapter.

- **Infliximab (Remicade)** in 1998. This is a monoclonal antibody, human IgGIK engrafted on murine Fg region. This antibody is produced in a murine myeloma cell line transfected with cloned DNA coding for cA2 and then purified. The cA2 antibody has a high affinity for soluble and membranous bound TNF-α this has a half-life of 7 to 10 days.
- **Etanercept (Enbrel)** was introduced in 1999. Dimeric fusion constrict that links two p75 (type T1) TNF receptors to the Fe portion to the IgG1. The drug has a long half-life. Produced in recombinant DNA technology in Chinese hamster ovary cells.

Enbrel inhibits TNF-α and lymphotoxin a to TNF receptors. Half-life 120 hours and does not lyse TNF-α expressing cells.

- **Adalimumab (Humira)** Introduced in 2002. Is a fully human IgG anti-TNF-α monoclonal antibody. Produced by phage display. Binds circulating and cell bound TNF-α and blocks inner action with P55 and P75 receptors. Does not interact with lymphotoxin TNF-b. It induces cell lyses of TNF expressing cells. Half-life 10 to 20 days.

These represent not only the beginning of the new biological and immunological era of rheumatology but also the understanding the pathology and management of arthritis.

THEN THERE ARE THOSE OTHER AUTOIMMUNE DISEASES

One might ask why so much space was given to Autoimmune Diseases [not AIDs, that title's been preempted by Acquired Immune Deficiency Syndrome [AIDS-HIV]. A listing of many such diseases are catalogued below. The reader might question why the author considers this recent work in Rheumatology is pointing a path to closing Pandora's Box of Diseases. Well, there are two reasons: the first is that recent Rheumatological work on halting the body's improperly produced antibodies and the recent development of drugs like Rituxan for Cancer generate an implication that we are on the way in one autoimmunity case in stopping antibodies from attacking good cells and in the second forcing antibodies to attack bad cells.

The second reason for this author's hopeful hypothesis is that Rheumatoid Arthritis is just one of many autoimmune disorders and solving one points the road to solving all. Autoimmune disorders can be broken down into Systemic and Organ-specific. Examples of organ-specific are Addison's, which attack the Adrenal Cortex; Graves, which attack the Thyroid, and Myasthenia Gravis, which attacks neuromuscular cell. Systemic examples include Lupus Erythematosus, and Arthritis.

So here is our list of those other considered disorders:
- Acute Disseminated Encephalomyelitis
- Addison's disease
- Ankylosing Spondylitis
- Antiphospholipid antibody syndrome
- Aplastic anemia
- Autoimmune hepatitis
- Coeliac disease

- Crohn's disease
- Diabetes mellitus
- Goodpasture's syndrome
- Graves disease
- Guillain-Barré syndrome
- Hashimoto's disease
- Lupus Erythematosus
- Multiple sclerosis
- Myasthenia gravis
- Opsoclonus myoclonus syndrome
- Optic neuritis
- Ord's thyroiditis
- Pemphigus
- Pernicious Anemia
- Polyarthritis
- Primary biliary cirrhosis
- Rheumatoid Arthritis
- Reiter's syndrome
- Sjögren's syndrome
- Takayasu's Arteritis
- Temporal arthritis
- Warm autoimmune hemolytic anemia
- Wegener's granulomatosis

A final thought after perusing this list allows one to wonder just what and where is the indicator or director mechanism in the immune system that decides which tissue to attack.

CHAPTER 4
MODERN CONCEPTS ABOUT INFLAMMATORY ARTHRITIS

As is inferred from the last section of Chapter 3, a great Rheumatologic advance has just been taken with the development of biologic drugs that bind themselves to certain autoimmune cells that the body mistakenly produced to destroy certain of its own body parts. On binding to those autoimmune cells, they are inactivated.

We now are approaching a stage in the management of Rheumatoid (Inflammatory) Arthritis that surpasses our earlier hopeful imaginings. The future has arrived, and the possibilities of reverse, or at least stopping the progress of Rheumatoid (Inflammatory) Arthritis are at a new height. This represents new vistas into projecting TNF-α (Tumor necrosis factor- alpha) drugs in managing many other medical diseases. They further offer potential elimination of all the devastation of inflammatory so-called autoimmune disease.

The future in managing arthritis invites thoughts of complete control and management of all phases of the disease. Starting with a supposition that the primary tissue instituting the damage is the synovium, the fundamental management should be directed at the synovial tissue. Early consideration of the joint destruction by the synovial tissue with local physically eroding of cartilage, it had all the appearance of a local malignancy. As more instances of joint problems appeared, it became obvious that mild Inflammatory Arthritis was a common phenomenon. It was not unusual for this to involve limited joint areas. In time, with greater clinical observational-data in hand, an acceptable conclusion surfaced that this mild inflammatory state could well be a precursor to degenerative joint disease. This was most obvious when completely damaged knees were observed in comparison to normal hips, or their contrary. An inference could be taken that a majority of the problem in degenerative joint disease was originating in the diseased synovium. It was the synovium that was a major contributor to selective cartilage degeneration! Even with this clue, determining the actual cause of Inflammatory Arthritis still eluded us.

Now there's clinical evidence demonstrating how the synovium manifests itself in Rheumatoid (Inflammatory) Arthritis, and that it's initiated by lymphocytes localized in synovial tissue. When these lymphocytes are activated, they first cause pain in and swelling of the synovium and then, joint- damage. These lymphocytes produce cytokines, which are protein mediators that:

- Initiate inflammation,
- Attract other immune cells to the site,
- Activate resident cells,
- Cause excess synovial fluid production.

The T-cells arrive through a complex process that mediates passage through the vascular endothelium into the synovial tissue. In this process, T-cells are attached to the vessel lumen via surface molecules that recognize adhesion molecules expressed on endothelial cells. Several interactions involving distinct pairs of adhesion molecules ultimately result in the localization of T-cells to synovial tissue.[2]

Having learned and understood the importance of the synovium, allows us to reassess past treatment in accord with the great chemical advances at our disposal today. All past treatment was directed towards decreasing swelling and at clearly inflamed synovial tissues. We had a rudimentary knowledge of its destructive nature, and none about the agents involved in the attack on that tissue. All that was clearly understood was that treatment was critically needed (something we have understood from 550 BC to 1950 AD).

Unfortunately, in those three millennia before Cortisone, we had only Aspirin to lower the pain. With so much unrelieved suffering, it is no wonder that the door opened to every well-intentioned thinker, and to every profit-minded quack came promoting his personal cure. Crackpots, dream faddist, alchemists, mavens, gurus, all took a fling. Recent ones were to name a few:

- Herbology, now called Alternative Medicine
- Green Druggists;
- Exercise;
- Acupuncture
- India's Ayurvedric;
- Homeopathy;
- Orgonomy;
- Dianetics;
- Yoga and Massage;

---

[2] "Rheumatoid Arthritis—A Molecular Understanding": J. Bruce Smith MD, and Mark K. Haynes PhD Ann Intern Med. 2002; 136, 908-922. www.annals.org

- Osteopathy and Chiropractic;
- China's Chui Dan Wha;
- Japans Shiatsu;
- Yin-yang balance;
- Natural Oils;
- Vegans and Biodynamic Farming;
- Kellogg's Battle Creek Sanatorium cereals.

Rather than just presenting a list, perhaps some of the most popular ones in American should be addressed a bit more:

HOW ABOUT EXERCISE?

Exercise, especially swimming[4], alleviates the pain associated with arthritis but few claim it to be curative.

BALANCING YOUR LIFE FORCE?

Western Orgonomy, Japanese Shiaatsu, India's Ayurvedric, and China's Chui Dan Wha [which balances the body's five forces (going the old Greeks one better) of Wood Fire Metal Water and Earth to get a stable Qi] have only anecdotal cures. Chinese-American clinics fare no better.

HOW ABOUT ACUPUNCTURE?

Acupuncture does sometimes relieve symptoms [of almost anything] but a five hundred-page book teaching the details of needling patients has written of only two RA case cures, mild ones at that improved.[4]

SOME FOODS TRIGGER RA?

Authors have become wealthy writing how certain foods like corn and its products [as well as milk products from skim to cheese]; Meats [beef, pork, chicken, turkey, llama, fish]; Wheat, [oats, rye]; Eggs; Citrus fruits; Potatoes; Tomatoes; Nuts; and/or Coffee either aggravate or trigger arthritic symptoms in some patients. Such allergies can be demonstrated, but are any of them a cause of RA? Not likely, or is it an effect from the antibody activity? Perhaps, or is it just an allergy that the body has and when RA comes, it finds a new attack port? Not that likely either, but one reality is that staying away from every food that gives the slightest indication of being harmful, doesn't cure arthritis: that fact you can take to a hospital bed, not to the bank. Liking the Vegan lifestyle or eating only foods from Biodynamic farms fit the same bill.

---

[3] Pain Free Arthritis Dverla Borshran 1978

[4] Esther, a 75-year-old retired nurse had severe arthritis and, after a year of treatment, she was free of pain and had recovered use of her joints and limbs with no recurrence for 15 years.

Jeanne Forsmith age 74 reports, "I couldn't use my fingers much. After a treatment I could open a jar again, I hadn't dome that for a long time".

Perhaps someday the five basic foods of Carlton Fredricks: Blackstrap molasses; Wheat germ; Brewers yeast; cottage cheese, and pumpernickel; will again be added onto the RA cure bandwagon.

HERBS or OILS WORK?

Some of the herbs listed are:

Some idiosyncratic hers are: Alfalfa; arnica; Bee venom; Devil's claw; Fecergew; Ginger; Fiaicum; Meadowsweet; Shark cartilage; White willow-bark; Mertex origini root; Chinshe root; Chinese mimosa-bark; Evening primrose; Black current; Mugwort; Tatswallia; Googool; Turmeric; Cinnamon; Duckvean; Chinese Skullcap; Mexican wildrun; VTVola; Ahwaganda; Sarsaparilla; Black walnut leaf, Chinese ginseng-root; Willow root; Knuckle root; Chinese Sissacue; Hawthorn berries; Chinese sterallax; Licorice; Kirkumin; Korean ginseng; Siberian ginseng . . . All herb gurus make an admonition that a herb doesn't cure everyone so the individual must experiment on all of them = trying each for a few weeks at a time - and then try combinations of those that seemed most effective.

Europeans and Americans tend to focus in on using oils like careen oil, mustard oil, ginger oil, and castor oil. Of course, the tasty oil used for popcorn as well as safflower, sunflower, and cottonseed oil are not listed.

MEDICAL CULTS, QUACKS, AND FADDISTS

They exist. It's best to ignore them unless your money bucket's too heavy. As will be discussed in far more substantial detail in the next dozen chapters, we Rheumatologists and our Pharmaceutical companies are not without error, some of them continuing and some under development.

In the medical field we thought, for a time, we'd stumbled across an all-purpose cure: the steroid called Cortisone. After their fashion, steroids and all nonsteroidal agents worked for a while. Originally, it was considered dangerous to inject steroids but recently their injection into the joint is understood to be effective and potentially articular-cartilage-saving. Now that we know inflamed synovium produces the cytokines, Interleukin-1 and tumor-necrosis-factor-alpha (TNF-α), which destroy cartilage. Suppression of inflammation, even if non-specific does protect cartilage. In not recognizing this, lay one of the multiplicative misconception-examples in past treatments.

Putting aside for a while, all we have learned about Rheumatology's grand new string of drugs, the detailed knowledge about the workings of immune system, there's a basic admission it has to make: The specific cause stimulating synovium inflammation in Rheumatoid

Arthritis is unknown. Until that's definitively learned, it's critical that we continue concentrating on the synovium. There's now definitive evidence that the inflamed synovium is the joint's prime factor in bringing articular cartilage damage. This mandates definitive and specific treatment even for any minor trauma that might incite inflammation, since it is now known that synovial molecular substances produce cartilage damage.

IT IS IMPERATIVE THAT SOME NEW CONCLUSIONS
BE BROUGHT FORTH REGARDING DJD

As was hinted at above, it was once considered that stress, and wear-and-tear were prime inciting factors in degenerative joint disease. Another commonly considered cause of degenerative joint disease is regarded as metabolic or genetic-based abnormal cartilage-integrity; that must be set aside with athletic-trauma. A continual assessment of late stage degenerative joints demonstrates degenerative joint disease isn't systemic. It generally involves isolated regions like hips and knees. If Degenerative Joint Disease is to be represented as a cartilage disease, some correlation with generalized cartilage degeneration should be demonstrated. In depth clinical manifestation suggests that DJD results after the earlier continually inflamed synovium was the predecessor, with that minimal degree of inflammation ultimately causing cartilage damage.

In degenerative joint disease [DJD], it is important to pay attention to inflammation of synovial tissue. Even at its earliest and minimalist stage, clinical evidence puts forward the significance of synovial inflammation. It's now known that cytokine substances produce the harmful inflammation in synovial tissue of the joint to enhance cartilage-damage. This knowledge alters the old ideas as to the primary cause of DJD. Consideration should now be given to what slow, progressive damage over years can do to the articular cartilage, especially when there is secondary synovial inflammation. A joint that has a continually inflamed synovium, no matter what the cause, will result in cartilage damage, and finally in DJD. Speeding up and adding to the severity of this sequence could be increases in or additional minor trauma causing sustained or increased synovial inflammation, constant bombardment of damaging elements to the cartilage.

A clinically demonstrated cause of cartilage damage offers greater evidence to the inflammatory origin of DJD. Recent molecular immunology points to the cytokines produced from diseased inflamed synovia; these are targeted by treatment directed at TNF-α and

Interleukin-1 [IL-1]. Soon, we should have a better and more specific approach to these and other substances that block the synovial-inflammatory, articular-cartilage-destructive process. We can only wonder as to what could be safely done once there is an agent that can be directly injected into an early-inflamed joint so as to retard the cartilage damage. This thinking is about a still mythical substance, which would be locally harmless, able to be injectable into the joint. It would thereby be easily monitored clinically to observe the result from decreasing the synovial inflammation. Future management of this sort could restrain the synovium from damaging cartilage. This and mild suppressive immunological agents could prevent ultimate disability, and cartilage damage, thereby altering the end-stage plight of degenerative joint damage.

With this knowledge and conceptual clinical observations, one can surmise interesting and very positive conclusions. With very early diagnosis and management of minor inflammation of joints osteoarthritis could result in preventing joint replacements? Many a surgeon would certainly consider this imaginatively hypothetical, if the disease is primarily one of cartilage. If DJD and cartilage damage is the result of the concept suggested here, then the cartilage can be protected, and joint replacements go the way of other surgical procedures.

Hypothetical is defined as assumed or proposed for further investigation. This theory is just so and will, as we progress, be described more fully.

Great strides will be made when we can inject into inflamed joints an agent that will bind TNF-α and IL-1. The ability to place the most effective agent directly at the problem's origin, thereby avoiding systemic administration will move us even closer to a cure. If early treatment of DJD by this specific joint injection of this anti-TNF-α agent is effective, most other drugs and treatments are eliminated. The effect of other systemic treatments can affect the system itself. Drug metabolism may change and alter any drugs chemical state as it is absorbed through the GI tract and liver while also binding with certain proteins in the circulatory system. The potential effects of drugs under these circumstances remain obscure part of drug treatment, and what effect metabolism has on the anti-TNF-α agents is yet to be clinically understood. This idea document's the final chapter [13] and will illuminate how far along such exploratory management has progressed, and the positive effect from it.

It was once considered that injecting steroids into joints was highly dangerous. Early teaching stated that local joint injection of steroid was itself damaging. This condition never clinically materialized. Long-standing procedural use of joint steroid injection was not harmful; it proved extremely helpful in decreasing synovial inflammation, and in maintaining joint functional capability. When one now understands the damage the cytokine substances in inflamed joints inflict, one realizes that the concept propagated about steroid joint injections was another misguided guess. Local joint injection treatment of an inflamed joint is most probably the best acute temporary treatment available. With new, specific agents being available, the dynamics in treating synovial inflammation will be totally changed. There is certain clinical evidence that such potential future treatment may truly save the articular cartilage, and offer new management programs for DJD by preventing cartilage loss.

The broad perspective of this very common joint disease spectrum with synovial involvement, and progression to cartilage damage, our reconsideration can then ask 'What is osteoarthritis'? The contrary concept is that DJD was a cartilage integrity disease. This can be the case for inherently deficient cartilage as well but, with the wide areas involved, isolated joints and asymmetry of osteoarthritis, doubt arises. Isolated joint disease and asymmetry can be explained by trauma, but cannot be explained on inherent primary-cartilage disease. That provides a different understanding for a possible mechanism of osteoarthritis. Whatever the inciting cause, one focuses on why is certain cartilage destroyed and other areas remain intact, e.g., hips, or knees can be damaged, with other joints being spared? This suggests isolated synovial inflammation. This situation could be the result of low grade, isolated, asymmetrical Inflammatory Arthritis, minimal trauma, or inclusion of other unknown factors resulting in synovitis with resultant cartilage damage and osteoarthritis, as is frequently mentioned.

Another possible hypothesis could be that there's a synergy between synovium and cartilage. It's biochemically evident that a diseased synovium contains substances that damage cartilage. The presence of degenerated cartilage was formerly considered that damaged cartilage causes the synovial inflammation: today's precise is the opposite.

A CLINICAL ANALOGY

Something very analogous to the previous situation occurs in the kidney with anemia. Renal failure produces anemia as the kidney decreases its production of the hormone that stimulates blood production, Erythropoietin. Anemia in turn decreases the renal function and the production of

Erythropoietin. Decreased red cell production decreases circulation to the kidney, which causes a further decrease in Erythropoietin and this caused further anemia. A circular 'Catch 21'[5].

A similar situation could exist within the joint between synovial tissue and cartilage. The degraded or injured cartilage creates abnormal joint function irritating the synovial tissue that causes the inflammation of the synovium. Within inflamed synovial tissue immune T-cells are present to produce cytokines that damage cartilage. That inflamed synovial tissue full of these immune cells now results in further cartilage damage. This circular circumstance results in the joint, as is analogous to the kidney Erythropoietin/anemia, circularity: each mis-feeding on the other. In this example, trauma to cartilage – be it micro or macro - and synovial inflammation - known or unknown - cause of primary inflammation would result in DJD not due to any inherent cartilage defect. This hypothesis adds an entirely different dimension to theorizing about the cause of degenerative joint disease. This theory offers more supports to the finding of asymmetry in DJD rather than it being a primary cartilage disease. It also adds new consideration as to treatment of this disease.

This clinical consideration of the concept of synovial tissue being a greater causation-element in DJD needs repeated reinforcement by further study and observation in order to be accepted. One may consider, upon scouring textbooks, that it borders on heresy to imply that synovial disease may be a cause of DJD. This unique characteristic of a mildly inflamed synovium as an implication in osteoarthritis implies DJD may not be a disease of intrinsic defective, or inferior cartilage, but the result of low grade, possibly long-standing synovitis. This may be an ultimately self-perpetuating perverted symbiosis between cartilage and synovium developing into osteoarthritis. There's much left to be understood now that advanced therapeutic drugs with their novel assault on cytokines impel us towards deeper contemplation concerning the cause minimal inflammation in the joint. The realization about the synovium being the source of damage from this inflamed tissue provides more possible causes of and treatments for degenerative joint disease.

---

[5]   Ancient Greek philosophers invented their 21st catch to wonder at: "If Darkness causes the Sun to rise, what causes Darkness to fall?" [or vice-versa]

THINKING FUTURISTICALLY

A spectacular advance worth hoping for would be to somehow measure serologically effects to detect early signs of synovial inflammation from *(TNF-α or other important cytokines)* by a simple blood test. That would assist in predicting potential cartilage damage. If one were able to measure early inflammation, the resulting treatment could possibly block and monitor the substances that were causing progressive cartilage damage. This situation could then eliminate osteoarthritis. Following acceptance to treat early synovial inflammation this way, osteoarthritis could be prevented and joint reconstruction would unnecessary.

Direct treatment of synovitis of all and any source must be directed at long-term suppression of the source of synovial inflammation. This demands major efforts for determining the cause of synovitis. What causes synovitis in general and why it persists, are questions provoking many and other challenging questions.

Asking *when* synovitis occurs rouses an idea that it may well be self-perpetuating. Just *what* is the source of autoimmunity and *how* does it come into existence? This adds importance to when the synovium becomes inflamed with a continuing production of cytokines and molecular substances what keeps the inflammation ongoing? Because of the very evident cellular changes that create molecular substances, which produce inflammation, even if the inciting agent diminishes, the cellular changes could establish that state of affairs as a lifelong one. It's clinically known that blocking these molecules (TNF-α) does not **stop** or cure the inflammatory disease. As we gradually learn more about the inflammatory process and become more skillful in advancing treatment – even while viewing it with a high index of suspicion – our certainty increases that damage and deformity shall someday become outdated horrors.

Rheumatoid Arthritis devastatingly damages joints, cartilage, ligaments, and structures proximate to the synovium. Even bone is in jeopardy from the substances produced by the specific T-cells in the synovial tissue. It's been demonstrated that Tumor-necrosis-factor-α and Interleukin-1 damage these structures directly. Now, with agents to block TNF-α and IL-1 in synovium, it's conceivable that damage could be avoided, provided the synovial inflammation is readily detected in an early or sub-clinical state. In situations where cartilage has already been damaged, transplant of autologus or cultivated cartilage will be another major advancement.

Rheumatology, more than any other field of medicine, is at the cutting edge of medical engineering. The most important ingredient is the ability to institute these new technological concepts and their resulting agents into treatment and management of the diseases. This will promote further searches for agents and into concepts, and an ability to access outcomes. From this, further ideas must result.

Rheumatology presently realizes that RA varies patient to patient. As drugs gain in ability to suppress the rheumatic activity, one develops a fine-tuning capability in employing the therapeutic effect of these agents. Clinical management of Inflammatory Arthritis will have to concentrate on the need to decrease the inflammation so as to suppress disease activity. With this will come greater alteration of drug doses and frequency of administration? Another such aspect needing consideration is the wide variety of drug combinations that may come to exist.

ADVANCES OF MANAGEMENT NEVER EVOLVE IN THE LABORATORY OR THE TEST TUBE! [6]

Advancement comes after long clinical use, and from experience with the various new drugs, present agents, and newer biological drugs still on someone's blackboard.

Projecting generations from now, one can estimate what might occur in evaluating and managing arthritic patients.

- Early detection of joint problems would center on determining the amount of synovial joint inflammation.
- The number of involved joints, swelling, determining quality, and quantity of synovitis that exists;
- Special serological tests to determine the volume of cytokines being produced and the quantity.
- A modernistic scan would become available to determine the degree of synovitis that exists.

From this scenario specialized tests lead to accurately customizing treatment. For each cytokine, would come a specific factor to block it. Any number of agents would be available to completely block the molecules created by the autoimmune cells causing the synovitis. In so doing, the underlying cartilage would be properly protected preventing premature degeneration of cartilage. This presupposes joints would be

---

[6] It was editorially orchestrated that this was a very cogent statement and should be highlighted

managed treated medically, and chemically protected through advanced immunological molecular pharmacology. The necessity for joint reconstruction and replacement would thankfully vanish.

This could lead to cellular advancement and management of most other autoimmune diseases. The consequence of assessing chemicals or pharmaceuticals in treatment, along with molecular advancement plus the involvement of genetic understanding will turn into reality what is now considered science fiction, just like traveling to the moon once was. Whether or when this will occur depends on winning the clinical freedom to utilize these and the upcoming drugs. If fear and timidity remain the side-effects of law firm litigation, this future management may not materialize until the litigators are handed their eternal reward.

THE NEW FUTURISTIC INCLUSION IN THIS MANUSCRIPT IS THE ATTACK WE MAKE ON THE NAME (RHEUMATOLOGY)

As advances in diagnosis and treatment have occurred, it's become evident that our venerable Rheumatological categorization and terminology is passé and on it's way to obsolescence. It's time to change the primary name of Rheumatoid Arthritis. *RHEUMATISM* is an ancient term of Greek derivation, which utilized the other ancient term mucous or (catarrh), which was depicted as an evil humor. This fourth body liqueur was felt to flow from the brain to the joints and other parts of the body. For centuries, the term rheumatism with its numerous verbally modified variations has spread to become amiable over-the-fence chitchat. This 5th century BC term is no longer suited to describing today's synovial inflammatory disease. Synovitis is becoming treatable and no longer carries an onus that Rheumatism once bore as being 'incurable' and 'crippling'. With greater clinical knowledge, earlier diagnosis, and the pathophysiology known today, the term Rheumatoid Arthritis, or rheumatism is a misnomer and a humorous one. It's time to rename and reclassify so-called rheumatic diseases.

With definitive understanding of the anatomic and pathologic tissue changes, terminology should befit both clinical and pathologic. Moreover, the term *Rheumatoid Arthritis* is actually a severely damaged end-stage, term for describing an arthritic disease. It seems to be proclaiming that arthritis, already with such a wide variety of symmetrical polyarthritis of existing joint damage and pathologic changes, owns a poor prognosis. This is appropriate for only a very small number of diseased individuals. The term, Rheumatoid Arthritis, is not appropriate for an individual of any age with mild synovitis, and with stiffness of the neck, shoulders, multiple joints, fatigue, and general aches and muscle stiffness.

This is not an unusual complaint being presented to a general practitioner who then off-handedly labels it as just arthritis that happens to old men; just take an aspirin. Following a real diagnosis, a close examination and further investigation of these symptoms could reveal slight tenderness and synovial swelling of the knees and mild tenderness of the metacarpal phalangeal areas and other symptomatic areas. With these definite and subtle findings, the diagnosis 'early rheumatoid' is the most befitting with a misleadingly inappropriate connotation. This brief illustration, of which there are many variations, tells why a pathological and anatomical descriptive diagnosis is more appropriate.

On examining clinical experience, the therapeutic modalities available, and a modern approach to treatment, it's clear that a better terminology is needed. Two very descriptive arthritic terms are: Osteoarthritis, and Degenerative Joint Disease. DJD implies a wearing down or deterioration of the joint, indicating an anatomical state of worn or damaged cartilage. This is a descriptive term anatomically focused on the tissue involved, but doesn't indicate any specific etiology or cause, making it a perfectly adequate diagnostic term.

Rheumatism or Rheumatoid Arthritis is not a suitable term for the modern constellation of symptomatic states of inflammatory joint diseases. It's time for a term more descriptive of pathophysiological problems occurring in affected joints. There is very specific evidence of what's occurring in diseased joints. In providing a sensible terminology, one must begin by considering the tissue involved—synovium and the management program. On accepting this concept, one must then consider the state and condition of synovial inflammation. For years it's been said that there are at least one hundred forms of arthritis. In actuality, there could be one or two forms of arthritis with one hundred ways of expressing this disease.

It's time for arthritis to acquire a better method of naming itself, and for categorizing Rheumatoid Arthritis. When used as a starting diagnosis, a patient having Rheumatoid Arthritis pictures a deformed individual with a terrible outcome. This RA condition comes in many persuasions. The name gives no clues as to its state or existing condition. The same situation existed in diabetes, which was truly generic for various kinds of the disease. Presently when one hears Type I or Type II diabetes, it has a definite clinical connotation. It's time for rheumatology to change the implication of Rheumatoid Arthritis into more meaningful and descriptive terms.

Rheumatoid Arthritis carries a bad connotation with little insight into or information about its state, and it isn't cognitive to individual patients.

It would be better described as
INFLAMMATORY SYNOVIAL ARTHRITIS and could be classified as follows:

Inflammatory Synovial Arthritis Class I.

In Class I, the patient provides
- A history of joint pain, stiffness, and/or fatigue with few or multiple joints.
- Critical examination reveals clinically detected swelling of the synovium in one or more joints.
- All other tests and findings are usually normal.

Inflammatory Synovial Arthritis Class II.

Class II is associated with
- Morning stiffness, joint pain, and stuffiness in one or multiple joints;
- Easily perceptible synovitis clinically noted and is so-designated by the patient.
- There can be joint effusion with this stage of arthritis.
- Clinical evidence of joint pain and swelling is easily detected.
- X-ray and laboratory evaluation, other than Sedimentation Rate may be normal.

Inflammatory Synovial Arthritis Class III.

At this stage Class III,
- All of the other findings are present but in a more aggressive state.
- X-rays will show changes of erosions.
- Abnormal laboratory test may be involved to assist in confirmatory evidence.
- Minimal joint deformity may be seen.
- Perhaps there is: slight interosseous; atrophy; and nodules.
- Dropped metatarsal heads.
- Slightly limited range of motion of the involved joints.

Inflammatory Synovial Arthritis Class IV.

This stage Class IV has
- All of the previous mentioned historical and physical findings,
- Obvious physical deformity of joints,
- As well as the entire classical findings of late disease.
- Evidence of joint replacement have occurred.

Further inclusion into the categorization could be the stages of treatment, which would be of greater assistance in our modern coding of the disease.

Such diagnostic re-labeling allows tailoring condition of the arthritis and management to more descriptive terms. The advent of biological drugs directed with specificity at the inflammatory tissue in this arthritis, illustrates that a more modern terminology is necessary. New terminology adds ease of description to the stage of the arthritis. It promotes greater understanding for patients as to the disease process. It provides more enlightened information in transcribing and transmitting data about the arthritis. The term Rheumatoid Arthritis alone has such a broad reference and poor connotation as to the stage of the disease and its severity. A modern alteration in terminology is long overdue and warranted.

The final and most important element in new stage terminology would be the ability to use these descriptive anatomical physiological stages in terminology to document the progression or regression of the disease. One could determine if the disease is advancing or being held in check, or improving - especially in assessing present and future drugs. We truly don't have such ability with the criteria available today.

We had stated that arthritis, as a disease, and Rheumatology, as a specialty, is at the cutting edge of medicine, providing a grand vista for its management future: one approaching a cure for this disease that fifty years ago was described as crippling and incurable. Rheumatology is not only at arthritis' end but also at the beginning of autoimmune diseases' end.

CHAPTER 5
HISTORY AND EXAMINATION IN ARTHRITIS

*T*extbook descriptions are simplistic and stereotypical at best. One must learn and comprehend the disease of Rheumatoid Arthritis from patients rather than anecdotal historical sketches. The history of the disease is the rheumatologist's most valuable tool. The clinicians obvious action is asking which joints are involved. In interviewing the patient, a series of critical questions are put forward in a variety of sometimes-redundant-seeming repetitions. However, a resonance of redundancy bemuses a patient, answering these questions cannot be stressed enough. Questioning is to be continued, albeit repetitiously, until no further information can be uncovered regarding the character of the symptoms and joints activities.

The very first and rudimentary approach of any present joint symptom or complaint must begin with these following questions:

- How long has the joint or joints been symptomatic in this present episode?
- How long has one had pain or swelling in the joint or joints?
- Specifically which joints are involved?
- Is it the first time these joints have been swollen and painful?
- If not, when was the first time? Was it one of a series of flares, and how often did it occur?
- How did the condition begin?
- Carefully describe a typical attack and how it occurred.
- Was it sudden, slow?
- How long did it last where and which joints were involved and how long?
- How many episodes over the years, and how many years?
- How have you treated or handled these flare-ups of joint attacks of pain and swelling?
- What medical or other treatments have you had in the past?
- What are you doing now to treat the present joint problems?
- Are you presently stiff on arising in the morning?
- Are your joints swollen? If so, which ones?
- What aggravates this present condition and how are you at present?
- What are you doing to treat the condition at this time?
- Describe how you feel now, and how did you feel this morning?
- Presently, which joints are most symptomatic, and what did you take today?

- What do you think is wrong?
- What is your diagnosis?
- Do you have any questions before I begin the physical examination?

This series of questions and a few more as the encounter proceeds reveals more about the disease than any area of the evaluation. Specifically one must focus on how the joint pain, swelling, and inflammation has progressed and acted. After concluding this series of questions, observing the patient, and completing a good physical and joint examination, the diagnosis of Rheumatoid Arthritis is made with almost complete certitude. The examination follows, but the concluding, definitive part of evaluating arthritis takes place during the follow-up time. This is truly how one learns about the individual's unique form of arthritis

ARTHRITIS EXAMINATION JOINT BY JOINT

Joint examination is described in numerous textbooks, monographs, and pamphlets, but each physician and rheumatologist develops an individual technique. The examination routine helps in joint diagnostics:

- Begin with *inspection* of the joints while visualizing joint motions; these are foremost damage indicators as the individual moves in the office, examining room, walks and removes clothing. This is done at the beginning as well as during the examination.
- Moving the arms over the head and behind the back reveals a great deal about the shoulders.
- Having the patient attempt to squat down, even holding on to a chair, discloses information about hips and knees.
- How far one can bend forward, assisted or unassisted, provides information about back and spine.
- Simply observing the limitation from pain involved in the examination and general movement is part of the examination.
- All the joints are then felt and put through a full examination regarding range of motion. From these simple functions, one is able to observe
- The degree of swelling in a joint.
- How thick and swollen the synovium may be.
- How painful, the degree of limited function, and
- If deformity and loss of function exists.

The next step is to determine how many joints are involved, to what degree, and how limited is their function. The loss of function is determined by attempting to discern if the loss is primarily from joint swelling and pain, or if the mechanical loss is the result of earlier severe damage to the joint with loss of cartilage.

Examination of the hands and wrist reveal a great deal. Wrists and hands possess groups of joints. Starting with the *wrist:* by feeling these joints, one can determine if there's any swelling of the synovial tissue. Along the surface of the wrist - on the side of the fifth finger, there is an indentation where the hand joins the bones of the forearm. As swelling ensues, the indentation disappears since the synovium bulges out from this area. This is characteristic of rheumatoid changes at the wrist. In addition, by just gently placing fingers and thumb on the patient's wrist, one feels warmth and thickness that can demonstrate synovial swelling and thickening. This, along with flexing down and extending up the wrist, will determine the range of motion in the wrist joint. In severe involvement, it can be markedly restricted. Tapping on the inner surface can determine if there is pressure on the median nerve if tingling occurs in the thumb and first two fingers. This demonstrates the carpel tunnel syndrome.

Feeling - or palpating which is the medical term - the *metacarpal phalanges* joints (MCP joints) where the hand joins the fingers is next. These become thickened, swollen, and tender, growing limited in flexion and extension while opening the hand and making a fist. Just squeezing the examiner's fingers is a test of grip strength, which is greatly diminished when these joints are swollen and involved with arthritis.

Feeling and moving those finger-joints known as *proximal inter phalangeal joints* (PIP joints) and then the *distal interphalangeal* joints will reveal a great deal about the type of arthritis that's troubling the patient. The metacarpal phalangeal joints and the proximal interphalangeal joints are characteristically involved in Rheumatoid Arthritis. When long-standing, these are the joints that result in the characteristic changes of the drifting of the fingers laterally and the flipper appearance in severe deformity of a classic Rheumatoid Arthritis hand. In early or mild stages, all that must be perceived is a swelling and tenderness in these joint areas.

Distal interphalangeal joints - or DIP joints as they are anagram termed - are important - but usually overly influential in making a diagnosis. When these joints show deformity with hyperthropic changes, Heberdan labels them with the term described centuries ago, called Heberdan's nodes, and depicted as osteoarthritis. A much broader description of this will be written further on in this multi-thesis monograph and is of great interest today.

It's important to have the *patient discern for themselves the swelling and thickening* of the metacarpal phalangeal area and joints. Have the patient feel one set of joints and then feel the other with the second and third fingers. This is done by touching the metacarpal head with the thumb on the top of the hand and feeling the underside of the metacarpal phalangeal joint with the fingers. The patient is then asked if he feels the thickened, spongy sensation of the swelling of the joint and synovial tissue. Patients feel it, but have no concept of the quality or quantity of the swelling of the joint, the capsule, and synovial thickening. The patient is then instructed to do the same thing to the examiner's hand, and it allows them to realize how much tissue is between fingers and to the bones of the metacarpal phalangeal joints. In addition, if there is increased temperature, he is made to perceive the warmth of his joint area. From this, the patient learns self-examination and how to perceive joint inflammation before deformity has occurred.

Elbow joints, on being examined, easily reveal synovial swelling, and readily demonstrate lack of full flexion and full extension of the elbow, which is 180 degrees, and beyond. In addition, rotation of the elbow is also a function that is easily tested. These simple tests reveal elbow disease.

The *shoulder* usually does not easily exhibit changes visibly, but is most revealing while it is moving itself in a range of motion to determine pain, swelling, and synovial involvement. Not infrequently, one can easily visualize large quantities of synovial fluid accumulating in the shoulder joint; it is easily felt and can be removed to be examined for specific therapeutic purpose. Much pathology frequently exists in this joint, which needs critical consideration and examination, frequently exhibiting problems needed for diagnosis and treatment.

Neck and cervical spines may be involved in frequent complaints of headache at the base of the skull, with limited range of motion while turning the head, with extension or on looking-up. There are many delicate structures in the cervical spines, such as small nerve roots, muscles, and the cervical area of the spinal cord. Careful examination while placing the neck through a full range of motion may suggest a variety of potential abnormalities. A definitive method of determining the amount of involvement here is by physical or x-ray examination.

Feet are very similar to hands in Rheumatoid Arthritis and have the same revealing features during inspection and physical examination. In Rheumatoid Arthritis, arthritis of the feet has almost the same involvement as in the hands. Patients frequently disregard their feet. They don't consider them similar and minimize their involvement. The feet have the same number of joints but are shaped, positioned and function differently than the hand, although they may have the same pathological changes. One ought to remember that some people born without fingers have used their toes to write novels and paintings. Most often, individuals accept foot pain, and the feet are then treated by a variety of other modalities. Toes drift laterally, just as do diseased fingers. Joints lie between tarsal bones (compare with the carpal bones) and the tarsal bones (compare with the phalanges) making up the tarsal metatarsal joints which are frequently painful and thickened with synovial swelling as in other forms of Rheumatoid Arthritis. These joints are easily examined although frequently being ignored. Often, after examining this area and eliciting changes and abnormality, the patient then volunteers its pain involvement. This area is diagnostically revealing, but is an area that's often neglected other than by a podiatrist. Physical and simple x-ray examinations can frequently generate the most revealing information about Rheumatoid Arthritis and other arthritic conditions of the foot.

Ankles are easily evaluated for swelling, both visually and by palpating. Ankle range of motion is readily determined from a passive range of motion in all directions. Ankles consist of three main bones. Arthritis or other involvements can be easily determined by a physical examination.

Knees are the most cherished joints for the rheumatologist. It is the joint most easily examined, the joint most complained about, and amenable to treatment. Simple inspection of a standing patient reveals swelling in the knee joint. Often, the patient is not aware of the swelling or the amount of distinguishing synovial swelling and thickening that exists. An important maneuver, as mentioned, has the patient squat, and through that exercise he generally appreciates how badly the knee joint has swelled.

When lying down, it is not difficult to appreciate the amount of swelling present and to estimate the amount of synovial swelling, and synovial fluid present. With the patient's head to one's left, by placing the left hand on the knee above the patella, - the knee cap - and the right hand below, one can distinguish the amount of swelling in the entire knee joint. Now, with the right hand placed firmly behind the knee, and the left hand compressing the patella, one can feel floating or ballott against the upper joint end of the tibia. Ballotting the patella illustrates the presence of synovial or other joint fluid. This allows one to ascertain the quantity of synovial fluid in that joint.

Warmth is easily detected. That's another important circumstance to have demonstrated to patients. Allow them to place their hand firmly but gently on the involved joint and compare it with the other joint with the same hand, allowing them to self-experience the warmth, thickening, and swelling. The knee joint is then carefully extended to its fullest to see if there is any hyperextension beyond 180 degrees. There is normally a slight amount of hyperextension of the knee, as in the elbow. On careful flexion, it is determined the range of motion there is and the amount of resistance and pain to 90 degrees flexion or beyond.

Holding the leg above the knee and gently moving it laterally and medially, one can detect if there is good or poor stability of the joints from its support ligaments. If there is minimal swelling and heat in one knee in contrast to the other, the patient occasionally is not fully aware of this. Next, place both hands on the knee with the fingers of one hand behind the knee. The space behind the knee is called the popliteal space. With the hand held behind the knee, one effortlessly feels thickening of the synovial tissue pouching out behind the knee. This can be easily compared to the untouched knee. In more severe instances, a large amount of swelling and fluid can be felt; this is referred to as a 'Baker's Cyst'. This area can be easily palpated and treated. This will be discussed in a later more-detailed chapter.

Hip examination is both crucial and simple. It is not uncommon for a patient to complain of 'hip pain' and place the hand on the cheek of the buttocks or the side of the pelvis, feeling assured they have a bad hip. Most often it is back pain, and its origin lies in the spine. Hip pain is primarily and basically located in the region of the groin. One of the most common complaints is losing easy rotation of the hip. The individual may not focus a great deal on pain but has a problem putting on socks or tying shoes. Hip pain frequently radiates to the knee and is often confused as being knee pain.

Hip examination is simply performed by having the patient lie on his back and flex the hip by bending the knee slightly in an upward, flexed position. Then, while in that position, the leg is rotated outwardly with the heel of the examined leg placed on the knee of the other leg, and then rotated in the other inward position. If the hip rotates freely in that manner without pain, there is no disease of the hip joint. Free movement action provides much information about the state of the hip. Finally, one can lay the patient on his side, upon the hip not to be examined, and then stretch the leg back to access the amount of hyperextension present. If this is all done freely, and without pain, then there is no hip arthritis of any amount. An x-ray for arthritis is not necessary when there is a normal range of hip motion on physical examination, but x-ray can confirm that the hip is not arthritic.

Physical examination of the _spine_ begins by observing posture and the gait. One most obvious postural gait revelation is from observing older men leaning slightly forward as they walk, as if walking into the wind. It is also the gait remembered only by the older readers – and trivia fans, which was the gait Groucho Marx mimicked.

That leaning foretells stiffening with slight flexion of the lumbar spines. This posture results from discomfort in an erect position and extension of the lumbar spines. The spine is not difficult to examine; one can assess forward bending or flexing to determine how mobile the spines are, and how far one can bend. Touching the toes or attempting to do so while observing the spines arching and movement, and the result of hyperextending backward reveals basic mobility, or immobility. Many times, the inflammatory process goes unnoticed or undiagnosed for many years on being confused as simple back problems, or with disc disease. Radiological findings are late in the Inflammatory Arthritis disease in the spine. It begins with changes or erosions and sclerosis of the sacroiliac joint and ultimately ends with calcification of the ligament and support structure. The characteristic appearance after long-standing disease in such as older men is a severe forward-bent. Occasionally it is seen in young men if the disease is aggressive and severe.

Following this history, taking an inspection, and examination of one with arthritis, it's not difficult to effectuate an impression or conclusion of what type or form of arthritis is present. After these elementary steps are taken, one proceeds further into a number of items in order to consider just what kind of arthritis is present and what treatment programs should be designed.

X-RAY DIAGNOSIS

In the recent past, liberal use of x-ray for evaluating arthritis resulted in studying subtle x-ray findings, hoping to find early changes that could help in diagnosing and treatment. Erosions of bone were its talking point. At surgery, it was noted that the synovial tissue, with consequent invasion and serious damage to joint structures, eroded cartilage and bone.

Radiologists then grew more interested in addressing any early erosive change, which might be seen on x-ray. Hands and feet were the most inspected areas since there the earliest changes were quite visible. These small joints revealed a great deal. The metatarsal heads (the so-called balls of the feet), the metacarpal heads (knuckles), and the carpal bones (wrist) were specific areas investigated by x-ray. It became more evident that, for years, these finding were being ignored and/or not noticed or appreciated.

In very careful inspection, especially under magnifying glass, one could detect small disruptions of the thin, bony cortex or edge that comprised the articular surface. As more study was undertaken, the x-ray changes noted became more intricate on being compared to the clinical picture. Demineralization was also considered in x-ray evaluation of Rheumatoid Arthritis. This demineralization finding was given greater consideration after the known devastation of osteoporosis, during the cortisone era. Loss of joint space was also noted on x-rays assessing that cartilage was damaged and lost. Synovial inflammation was bringing about various degrees of erosions. Rheumatologists now pride themselves on being able to evaluate early x-ray changes that most radiologists overlooked. They developed a finer grain of x-ray film to assess these early stages so that x-ray became a major test used by rheumatology. Skill in reading x-rays is now part of rheumatology training. X-rays of knees, hips, all the small joints, and the spine are now liberally used to evaluate arthritis. The field of rheumatology is gradually and continuously broadening.

CHAPTER 6

WHY MODERN THOUGHT DEEM TRADITIONAL ARTHRITIS NAMES NEED TO BE CHANGED

*T*he term *rheumatism* [7] was once the nomenclature for both a general, painful symptomatology of the musculoskeletal system, and a disease diagnosis. The word is derived from the Greek word *rheumatismos;* to designate the mucous (phlegm or catarrh)[8] as an evil humour thought to flow from the brain to the joints and other parts of the body. Today, the term rheumatism isn't found in the 12th Edition of *Primer on the Rheumatic Diseases* or in Barron's *Dictionary of Medical Terms.* Even the term 'rheumatic diseases' isn't defined in present literature; it remains a generic term for a wide variety of musculoskeletal diseases and has become the generic term for arthritis.

Any and all joints are subject to becoming arthritic. The degree and type of alteration to bone, cartilage, and synovium determines how a specific arthritic condition is defined. To simplify one form into degenerative arthritis is far too elementary, since that adjective implies a specific cause: wear-and-tear! Numerous diagnoses of rheumatic diseases are derived from a constellation of symptoms and areas involved and, over the years, specific terms have been attached to them as a diagnostic term. Medicine unfortunately has named disease by the end result and the havoc the disease has caused. In the final analysis, end-stage names are misleading and suggest grave and scary consequences. Such names as Rheumatoid Arthritis, Lupus, Scleroderma and more are examples.

WHAT IS RHEUMATOID (INFLAMMATORY) ARTHRITIS?
Rheumatoid (Inflammatory) Arthritis (RA) is primarily a disease of the synovial tissue. This prime tissue causes all the damage and destruction in the joints themselves. RA has, in most past and modern writings, been considered to be a deforming and crippling disease, which had been well described, way back in 1895, by Sr. William Osler. Since he wrote, we

---

[7]   *Hollander, Joseph in Arthritis and Allied conditions, Chapter I page 3*

[8]   *The Greeks considered there to be four humours controlling the body and they had to be maintained in strict equilibrium in the body to ensure health. The other three were yellow bile [urine], blood, and black bile [from the gall]. We might laugh at those old guys had our doctors not continued to practice even after the Renaissance - blood letting a century ago.*

have determined that synovial tissue can act in a wide variety of ways, and be present in many locations.

Rheumatoid Arthritis is generally considered a disease of multiple joints, but it can be a localized joint disease. As technology has evolved over the years, rheumatology diagnoses and treatments modalities have expanded along with biochemical understanding; considerations about the disease has altered a great deal. The addition of reconstructive surgery has eliminated an aspect of this disease that: it'll cripple you forever.

RA is a chronic, systemic, inflammatory disease that causes the synovial membranes to proliferate when inflamed and attacked by an influx of immune T-cells. It affects multiple body joints and generally is symmetrical. Being systemic, in a severe disease, there are at times many extra-articular RA features as well. It primarily is a mild disease but generally not recorded that way. Despite popularized beliefs, RA doesn't have the onerous connotation pictured in available writings: descriptions that, when an RA diagnosis is presented, the individual involved is generally devastated. The case normally being mild, any such connotation needs be dispelled quickly, then and there. The greatest percentage of RA cases is mild and treatable. While describing the disease, systemic elements are always included: neuropathy, scleritis, lymphadenopathy, pericarditis, splenomegaly, and arteritis, especially when the disease is very violent, but that's a rare form for RA these days.

In most cases, our literature describes RA as having remissions and exacerbations of the symptoms. Exacerbation means there are periods of time when the patient 'feels good' with the arthritis gone, and then times when the patient 'feels worse'. There will likely be times a patient with RA 'feels cured'. And there are patients that have had a complete remission. Treatment programs established by knowledgeable physicians and rheumatologists have been written in books and journals that lay out general management - almost in cook book fashion with a standard number of established drugs – stating that inflammatory Rheumatoid Arthritis will rarely 'go away'.

This also is a misconception continually propagated. The disease Rheumatoid Arthritis as described in all medical libraries is far different than what is clinically seen in a rheumatologist's office. RA can be mild but works individualistically upon every patient, since no two people, even if having the same anatomical structure, react biochemically or immunologically the same. Are there truly over one hundred kinds of arthritis or accurately over one hundred expressions of the same disease?

RA IS AN AUTOIMMUNE DISEASE

This medical book desires to present matters not written about in most standard texts and monographs. It's aimed at the larger number of patients with RA, a disease that can completely remit and sometimes never only to return, or return many years later wearing a different expression.

RA is considered an autoimmune disease in which the immune system is producing immune factors attacking ones own synovial tissue. Genetic factors may play a role in why this occurs in some individuals. The presence of an antibody (HLA-DRY antibody) in a significant number of RA patients with RA lends support to some degree of a genetic predisposition towards acquiring this disease. Rheumatoid Factor (RF), the antibody to an immune substance (IgG), was one of the early blood serum elements, which were considered its disease marker. Often and again, this has been searched for in tests to establish the diagnosis of RA. It's even stated to be present in 70% of cases. Most people waiting for these diagnostic blood serological tests will suffer for years undiagnosed while wasting elsewhere-needed money as well as years before their correct treatment commences. Too much attention has been paid to this specific antibody test, not for diagnosing the patient, just to help in finding the origin of RA.

High titers of RF written about are considered associated with more severe and active joint disease, having greater systemic involvement, and a poorer prognosis for remission. RA, as well as other autoimmune diseases, includes widespread immunologic and inflammatory alterations of connective tissue. Because the so-called autoimmune diseases share many clinical-findings, a differential diagnosis is often made difficult. Although the autoimmune disorders are considered acquired diseases, their causes usually cannot be determined. Systemic serological findings being too frequently relied upon don't correlate with the clinical picture. That's why these tests frighten individuals by what they have read on-line, or in books.

JUST HOW PREVALENT IS RA?

One or two percent of our general population is calculated to have arthritis. Years of clinical observation would reveal that this figure is far too small, especially since mild episodes of RA are not included. Females with RA outnumber males three to one. Onset of the disease in adults is reported to lie between the ages of 40 to 60; however, this is a meaningless statistic since RA can occur at any age. Acute cases have been diagnosed in the eightieth decade. Statistics are unimportant because there's no way of enumerating mild cases some of which are never treated.

ETIOLOGY

The etiology of RA remains unknown. Metabolic and nutritional factors, the endocrine system, geographic, psychological, and occupational data have been extensively studied with no conclusive findings. It now appears that an unknown antigen or agents, virus, chemical, genetics or a combination of them, may initiate an autoimmune response that results in RA. The disease acts like an infection on the system. Searching for some type of infection or post infection agent has been going on for years.

Rheumatoid Arthritis can affect many joints in the body, including knee, ankle, elbow, and wrist, and it is generally symmetrical. The joints having RA are usually tender, swollen, and will likely be demonstrating reduced motion. The basic key for all diagnosis and treatment in Inflammatory Arthritis (RA) is the synovial tissue. This synovial tissue - where the disease is – is focused on in recent age management of synovial joints.

SYNOVIAL JOINTS

A synovial joint has five basic components:
- Joint capsule is composed of two layers, an outer fibrous layer, and the inner synovium, called synovium membrane.
- Articular cartilage which has two important functions including: the ability to minimize friction and wear between two opposing joint surfaces during movement; and to dissipate forces on the joint over a wider area, thus decreasing stresses on the contacting joint surfaces.
- Synovial fluid, which bathes the joint. It contains hyaluronate (hyaluronic acid) and a glycoprotein called lubricin. Both are responsible for lubricating the joint. Synovial fluid is also the medium by which nutrients are carried to, and wastes carried from the avascular cartilage components of the joint.
- Subchondral bone is the ends of the long bones that form the synovial joints. It is a soft, spongy bone.
- Hyaline (articular) cartilage covers this bone and protects it. Except for the very ends of the bone, long bones are usually very strong.

In the course of a diseased joint, effusion and inflammation of the synovium occurs, producing a soft tissue swelling, that is to say: INFLAMMATORY ARTHRITIS. During an evaluation of the patient with RA, the inflamed synovial tissue can be easily detected.

After the disease has been present for years, (RA) demineralization of the bones forming the joint may show its effects. Early involvement at a minimal state, and through the progression, is associated with the common symptom of morning stiffness. Something that is always discussed in studies and textbooks that has import is the severity and duration of morning stiffness. Knowing about it is undoubtedly a helpful clinical tool

Disease symmetry is typically noted in joints among the following,

- Wrists, elbows, shoulders, knees which are the common large joints involved;
- Knuckles, (metacarpal carpel phalangeal joints – (MCP joints), which are the joints at the base of the fingers by the palm of the hand;
- Proximal interphalangeal joints (PIP joints) are the middle joints of the fingers;
- Hips, some areas of the spine, and sacroiliac joints are involved;
- Ankles and feet are most commonly involved;
- Metatarsal Phalangeal joints or (MTP joints) of the feet are comparable to the MCP joints of the hand are frequently involved.

Early in the disease, edema or swelling begins to be seen in the synovium with an influx of immune cells, and multiplication of synovial lining cells. This is what we call synovial tissue proliferation. This is clinically detected, and indicates where the treatment must be directed. As the disease progresses, the synovium may grow considerably larger eventually forming tissue called Pannus, destroying the joint. Pannus is now a term having limited used. Synovial tissue is the key to the structure that can be considered the most destructive element affecting joints in an RA patient. Further, it can destroy the soft subchondral bone once the articular cartilage protecting it is gone. This destruction is early seen on x-ray and termed erosions.

JOINT DAMAGE

The aggressive proliferation of the synovium causes destruction of bone eventually leading to laxity in tendons and ligaments. Under the strain of daily activities and other forces, these alterations in bone and joint structure result in the deformities frequently seen in patients with Rheumatoid Arthritis. As RA progresses with damage to articular cartilage, and with symptoms of inflammation, this compounds mechanical damage, as seen in degenerative joint disease.

Bone destruction occurs in regions where the hyaline cartilage is encroached on by the synovial lining. If the disease progresses to a more advanced stage, the articular cartilage may lose its dense structure, resulting in an inability to withstand normal forces placed on the joint. In advanced cases, muscle activity causes the bone-ends to compress together, causing further bone destruction. Further on, the disease can irreversibly change the structure and function of a joint to such a degree that other degenerative changes may occur, especially in weight bearing joints. Thus, joint destruction can progress to an extent that joint motion is significantly limited, and joints can become markedly unstable. It is the diseased synovial tissue that is the source of the damage to articular cartilage and compounded secondarily by trauma to the cartilage. Recently available agents are the exciting and dynamic biological elements that potentially shall prevent such devastation.

OSTEOARTHRITIS (DEGENERATIVE JOINT DISEASE)

Degenerative Joint Disease (Osteoarthritis, DJD): Osteoarthritis is described in all arthritis writings as a chronic disease causing deterioration of joint cartilage and formations of new bone (bone spurs) at the margins of the joints. Alternative names for this condition include:

- Hypertrophic Osteoarthritis;
- Osteoarthrosis;
- Degenerative Joint Disease, and DJD.

Cause and effect of Osteoarthritis will be presented with a unique clinical opinion. For most, the cause of osteoarthritis is the wearing out of metabolically inferior cartilage, which has resulted because of abnormal, genetic, chemical, and mechanical factors all taken into account, as they play roles in cartilage development and premature deterioration.

Osteoarthritis, the most common form of arthritis, is associated with the aging process. It may first appear in one's thirties or forties without symptoms; it is present in almost everyone by the age of seventy. Joint inflammation symptoms that appear in middle age (near fifty-five) may have unique circumstances as an underlying cause for this arthritis. DJD occurs equally in both sexes, however, after fifty-five its incidence is reported in most literature to be higher in women.

The cartilage of the affected joint is roughened, becoming worn and eroded as the disease progresses. The cartilage eventually wears completely away, so bone rubs on bone, usually with bony spurs develop around the joint. This represents the basic pathological description of osteoarthritis, as is described in literature of the last forty or fifty years or longer.

Systemic symptoms, sometimes associated with mild or severe Inflammatory Arthritis, are not commonly associated with osteoarthritis. The joints of the hands, fingers, hips, knees, great toe, or cervical and lumbar spine are commonly affected with both RA and DJD arthritis. The degeneration of the joint can occur from trauma to the joint, occupational overuse, obesity, or mal-alignment of the joints (for example being bow-legged, pigeon-toed, or knock-kneed). It can also occur from synovial inflammation.

Prevention frequently centers on weight reduction decreasing the risk of developing osteoarthritis on weight bearing joints. Since trauma is considered to play an etiological role, it too must be addressed as an important causative factor. Increased focus and interest in osteoarthritis has resulted in attentiveness to the joint architecture, symptoms, and function.

Diagnosing osteoarthritis is similar to all other rheumatic conditions. The history and physical findings with the appropriate use of x-rays to assist in determining structure and damage to a specific joint provides the necessary information. The specific joint involved, how, and where affected, along with physical appearance, is the basis in diagnosis of osteoarthritis.

What has been summarized is the actual canned teachings on DJD. Now it's time to move past traditional teachings of DJD, and give a modern consideration to the disease based on clinical experience.

Osteoarthritis is conventionally categorized as a developmental abnormality; a structural disease of articular cartilage. This conclusion has been espoused in all arthritis literature for years. With this as a cause, traumatic events are then bringing loss of surface articular cartilage in a wide variety of joints, and ultimately, wear-and-tear. The physiological structure of cartilage and its biochemical metabolism have been studied considerably in attempting to determine why and how it deteriorates. It isn't difficult to visualize the osteoarthritis that develops in an athlete's later years. They continually encounter trauma, damage, and frequent removal of injured cartilage segments. Impaired circulation to cartilage, especially in the hip, can be an underlying cause. Anything that embarrasses the cartilage such as trauma or inflammation can ultimately produce osteoarthritis. Under these criteria, it can often result as being considered a secondary phenomenon.

Many still consider osteoarthritis as a primary cartilage disease. The definition of osteoarthritis in the medical dictionary[8] states that it's the most common form of arthritis occurring in the aged, characterized by degenerative joint changes. Moskowitz[9] suggests that the term "Degenerative Joint Disease" may be more appropriate. More consideration of this disease is necessary because of its incidence and

---

8.
 Barron's Medical Guides, Dictionary of Medical Terms, Fourth Edition
9 Moskowitz, Roland W, *Arthritis and Allied Conditions*, Chapter 56, Clinical and Laboratory Findings in Osteoarthritis,

morbidity. A careful detailed clinical analysis of joint location and presentation needs further assessment before considering an underlying cause.

DJD, osteoarthritis is considered the most common form of arthritis. It will be contemplated here that it may really be a consequence of inflammatory joint disease. Textbooks refute this consideration, suggesting it may not be an inflammatory disease at all, but be better described as 'Degenerative Joint Disease.' As in most descriptions of this disease, many names and descriptions have evolved over the previous millennia. These fill rarely used texts with names, thankfully not known today. Much of it comes via the joints involved and the response of the affected tissues. Many of these so-called syndromes were named after their discoverers. Bone and cartilage characterize the descriptive clinical findings and also by our past pathology findings. Much of the time, the synovial tissue not being considered part of the osteoarthritis problem has been ignored. Something not part of a problem cannot be part of its solution. A recent example of the neglect, DJD has had in fundamental consideration of etiology is evident by the fact Edition 12 of the *"Primer of the Rheumatic Diseases"* published by the Arthritis Foundation is 680 pages and a scant 12 are related to DJD.

Unlike the traditional assertion, an alternate way to consider the disease osteoarthritis is to reflect on what is thought to be classic findings, i.e. hallmarks, of osteoarthritis [o.k. Degenerative Joint Disease], Heberdan's Nodes: hard bony spurs at the distal joints of the fingers. A foremost consideration is that Heberdan's Nodes are pathognomonic of DJD. Pathognomonic by definition is "a sign or symptom specific to, or characteristic of, a particular disease". These nodes are described as bony overgrowth or bony spurs involving the distal interphalangeal joints (DIP) of the hands. On appearance, they generally are symmetrical and involve most of the distal phalangeal joints. On examination, they are hard, bony overgrowths, and on x-ray analysis, they show bony spurs associated with loss of joint space, indicating loss of articular cartilage. At times, in the development of these nodes, they are described as end-stage Degenerative Joint Disease of the distal interphalangeal joints (DIP). As they evolve, they can grow to be quite tender with perceptual swelling.

These distal interphalangeal joints in this condition are associated with swelling, warmth, and occasionally have fluid within them. They even have out-pouching of the joint capsule with small nodes full of gelatinous fluid - similar to that found in ganglion cysts of the wrist or Baker's Cyst of the knee. These cysts are lined with synovial type tissue comprised of cells that produce a fluid similar to thick, gelatinous synovial fluid. This alone suggests more is occurring than 'Degenerating Cartilage'. Frequently, the proximal interphalangeal joints (PIP) of the hand are involved. When present, the appearance is in both sets of finger-joints, proximal and distal. On x-rays, both the proximal and distal interphalangeal joints reveal spurs and bony overgrowth along with loss of joint space due to loss of cartilage and erosions. This is now been labeled 'Erosive Osteoarthritis.'

This observation is the cause for creating the following didactic discourse concerning the pathology of Degenerative Joint Disease. First, there is its generally accepted primary cause, loss of cartilage from an intrinsic cartilage metabolic defect. It's too simplistic for this observer to conclude that it is the prime defect and the basic cause. When there is articular cartilage loss and erosions that results in a stimulation of bony overgrowth including spur formation, which is pathognomonic of DJD. How could this be a consequence of an intrinsic cartilage that's in such an insignificant isolated joint? These small joints show all the characteristics of larger joints that develop the same process as in knee and hip; the traditional conclusion is simply faulty metabolic articular cartilage where degeneration results from trauma (i.e., Degenerative Joint Disease). These similarly affected small finger joints have not been exposed to the trauma that weight bearing joints experience, but have the same pathology even though both are assigned the same cause: trauma and wear-and-tear in an inherently defective isolated cartilage of the finger joints alone. Such an apparently faulty conclusion raises suspicion regarding DJD's accepted causation.

A person of advanced age with moderate or severe knee or hip pain, whose x-rays show loss of joint space and spurs formation, is simply considered to have Degenerative Joint Disease. Concomitantly, it isn't unusual for other weight bearing joint groups not to be involved. For example, it is not unusual to see a pair of severely degenerative knees while the hips are normal, and visa versa. This creates problems with the supposition that DJD or osteoarthritis is primarily a disease of imperfect cartilage. If so, one must explain why the cartilage of the fingers not subjected to weight bearing or severe trauma, show findings similar to knees or hips that were subjected to these stresses.

A great deal of research still centers on studying aspects of Degenerative Joint Disease. All this effort remained centered on the cartilage, its structure, and metabolism. An earlier, the 11th Edition of *Primer on Rheumatic Diseases* published by the Arthritis Foundation contains more than five hundred pages with only two of them on osteoarthritis, epidemiology, pathology, and pathogenesis. Further meager discussions on the topic of DJD occurred but have resulted in no innovative concepts.

Much of its conception of osteoarthritis rests on stress and trauma. This undoubtedly is a factor, but after extensive consideration, one may be allowed deliberation to conclude that causation is not as narrow as generally presented. For most DJD cases - where more long-term comparison of clinical experience was compiled - the concept presented here ought to be given greater attention. The precursor to most DJD cases should be considering that of a smoldering, low-grade, clinical, or sub-clinical Inflammatory Arthritis.

Now that this notion has been broached, the attempt will be to take the idea further. The point has been reached when it's appropriate to give modern clinical deliberation to the diagnosis of DJD. When there is pain, soreness, and stiffness in joints especially with perceptible swelling, one must consider the structure of the joint and what mechanical causes, are creating the problem. Clinical joint abnormality obviously goes along with inflammation and the its symptomatic sequence. Modern arthritis management accentuates these different sequences of events, and it should be contemplated for osteoarthritis, or Degenerative Joint Disease. Injections of steroids into involved joints and the use of other anti-inflammatory agents are effective treatments. The more one evaluates, manages, and treats so-called typical-DJD, the easier it is to change our venerably ancient analyses relating effects to cause.

Beginning with the basic concept that as Rheumatoid Arthritis is a disease of synovial tissue, DJD is a disease of cartilage. Conceptually, this would indicate that there is a metabolic abnormality in the structure or cartilage makeup providing the premature or enhanced degeneration, or breakdown. As one inspects x-rays of degenerative joints, typically shows loss of joint space, spur formation, and underlying sclerotic bone. These are the hallmarks of progressive wear-and-tear with secondary new bone formation and some reshaping of the joint – all of this suggesting a slow progressive degradation beginning with the wearing down of the cartilage.

This has been the standard for contemplating and diagnosing DJD. Much research and effort has therefore been spent on studying cartilage, its make-up, and metabolism in order to determine just how this process comes about. As in Rheumatoid Arthritis, the synovial tissue and the inflammatory response is studied in detail to understand the disease and invent mechanisms to manage it. To treat and manage DJD better, study has been focused on the cartilage. However, we still have no real conclusive evidence regarding how and why the so-called autoimmune process commences in Rheumatoid Arthritis [or in any of the other autoimmune ailments]. The same is true about the cause for DJD if it has its origin in an inferior cartilage make up. It is even more puzzling and confusing when one ascribes DJD to simple wear-and-tear of cartilage.

There is no question that trauma is a major consideration in a great number of DJD causes. Today, most commonly often seen is knee damage and wear-and-tear from joint overuse. The modern vogues about knee damage are tearing of the medial meniscus and/or tearing of the anterior cruciate ligament. Without question such an injury to the knee will someday result in the development of DJD, but is that all there is to DJD? One major episode or many minor episodes undoubtedly produce and result in Degenerative Joint Disease of involved joints. This common phenomenon may have led to the consideration that DJD is simply trauma to the cartilage, and it alone is the background to DJD.

This period in rheumatology is one of being able to utilize a large number of agents in a variety of combinations to treat arthritis. Theorizing about what is the cause and the underlying problem of degenerative joint disease is intriguing. DJD is one of the most commonly seen conditions in women of almost any age: young, middle, or even older who are initially seen with mild pain, stiffness, and an almost imperceptible swelling of one or both knees. Evaluating and managing this condition over a number of years, the idea that this degenerative arthritis results by defective cartilage alone as a reasonable consideration in DJD may not be valid.

If perceptive low-grade inflammation compounded by excessive weight and/or mild trauma continues or persists, it undoubtedly will embarrass cartilage now or in the future. It's therefore not difficult to assume Degenerative Joint Disease will result. Since this condition of mild inflammatory synovitis can continue as a mild inflammatory process for years, and usually responds well to modalities discussed earlier. The concluding consideration therefore, concerning the eventual treatment of DJD, the treatment of mild inflammatory synovitis is to prevent the ultimate enhanced cartilage damage to the joint.

Going a step further, we can presumed if this early inflammatory state is neglected or ignored, the result may be precisely what is seen with classical DJD of the knees. As one labors with this assertion, the following results, an individual seen with the classical DJD gives some credence to the possibility that the precursor to the presenting condition of degenerative joint condition could have begun years earlier as a low-grade inflammatory process. Inflammation that is neither altered nor treated is why the damaged joint has arthritis. Additional support of this thesis is given by the fact that it's more common than not to see someone with degenerative joints in one area, while the other area of weight bearing joints are clinically normal. The most common areas are knees and hips. A patient can be seen with one or two degenerated hips and x-ray illustrates loss of joint space and sclerotic femoral head and acetabular component. From all appearances, one or both hips have totally worn out or completely degenerated. In that very description, the traditional assumption is that the cartilage gave way or degenerated due to defective cartilage, resulting in DJD of the hip.

If this is the conclusion, that there is, or was, inherent disease or weakness or fragility of the cartilage of these knee joints, or the hips as was illustrated, why then was it selective? Why were the other joints not provided with the same deficient cartilage or cartilage easily subjected to premature damage? The question then is if the hip cartilage degenerates why not the knees or visa versa? It's more common for one to see isolated Degenerative Joint Disease than a generalized degenerative joint condition. It is also common to see knees in a degenerative condition with normal hips,

Adding its weight to this thesis is clinical evidence that most Degenerative Joint Disease is the result of early Inflammatory Arthritis or secondary isolated trauma and not a basic intrinsic cartilage disease. It is common to find patients who have the obvious appearance of so-called Osteoarthritis-DJD of hands. These patients exhibit stiffened hands with hypertrophic changes of the metacarpal phalangeal joints, the proximal (PIP) and distal inter-phalangeal joints (DIP) on hands that are so stiff they cannot make a full fist, or completely flex all these joints. These aren't weight-bearing joints subject to the trauma like knees or hips and, at the same time, their knees and hips are perfectly normal. Therefore, if the entity described in the hands is DJD that implies the condition is an intrinsic disease of cartilage, if so why have the areas most subject to trauma been spared, or far less involved?

The conclusion would be that DJD which is modest or severe deformity and hypertrophic changes are secondary to a longstanding low-grade inflammatory synovitis resulting in weakening of the integrity of the cartilage. This use produces wear-and-tear on these joints, resulting in DJD. The other possibility is that isolated joint trauma causes the same sequence of anatomical event to result in DJD. This consequently suggests that there are these two causes of DJD as a secondary disease that now is existing as the primary disease we call DJD.

However, let's assume that low-grade Inflammatory Arthritis preceded the vast majority of DJD cases. The question still exists as to how much trauma it then takes to secondarily cause mild inflammation in a degenerated joint? Taking the question back to wear-and-tear and low-grade trauma, it still exists as a basic factor in DJD. This remains a difficult area to sort out in many a mind, but one thing that remains clear is an element of inflammation is almost always present in Degenerative Joint Disease at some time, providing much of the symptomatology accountable for its response to anti-inflammatory agents. In addition, there's no question that pain can come from existing mechanical damage alone.

Traditional treatment of osteoarthritis consists of intermittent joint injection with a long-acting steroid as in rheumatoid disease and, in most stages of DJD; the injected affected joint is as responsive as in typical Inflammatory Arthritis. Furthermore, oral NSAID's and analgesics are quite effective before the joint has fully deteriorated enough to require reconstructive replacement. Now modern molecular immunological findings suggest activity occurring in the synovial tissue can be a precursor to cartilage damage and degeneration. Further investigation and consideration of synovial inflammation and its potential cartilage damage provides unique decipherment to the cause of DJD.

Arthritis is a very dynamic disease with sometimes a violent appearance as with a severe Rheumatoid Arthritis patient. The osteoarthritis patient generally has a long, slowly developing condition. Osteoarthritis has so many appearances and presentations that it is easy to draw many conclusions as to some underlying cause. At times, one can be totally convinced that all DJD is nothing but secondary to underlying low-grade Inflammatory Arthritis and, at other times, be just as convinced that it appears to be a weakened form of a metabolically inferior state of the cartilage.

Many orthopedic surgeons are universally convinced that DJD is primarily a disease of cartilage, and this is difficult to refute that it is pure trauma. Rheumatologists, on the other hand, witness joint disease over longer periods, with much hands-on observation. They easily come to the conclusion that the primary underlying factor is more of a predisposition due to an early amount of Inflammatory Arthritis. This experience leads to another interesting observation.

Recent molecular and biological approaches to the treatment of Rheumatoid Arthritis and severe synovitis add further insight to this suggested concept for DJD causation. Information has arisen - from the development of new agents - that adds credence to this near heretical notion. Biochemical scientific studies on newly produced specific pharmaceutical agents possess special anti-inflammatory action. They are molecularly active in blocking substances being produced by immune cells within the inflamed synovium; those immune cells are producing molecules that directly damage cartilage.

Add trauma to this sequence, and the result, in time, is DJD.

INFLAMMATION AND DJD

While directing a great deal of attention toward the inflammatory aspect of arthritis, osteoarthritis took on another dimension. Osteoarthritis is customarily categorized in all arthritic literature as a primary developmental abnormality and structural disease of cartilage. This consideration was complemented by x-ray analysis showing loss of joint space and articular cartilage with secondary hypertrophic spur and sclerotic bone formation. This resulted in the accepted fact that osteoarthritis is primarily a disease of cartilage whose premature degeneration was principally, or secondarily, due to trauma.

Inflammation in osteoarthritis exists and must provoke consideration as to its etiology. The joints diagnosed as osteoarthritic are painful, slightly deformed, and frequently demonstrated clinical inflammation in the condition, at some point. Steroids, locally injected into the involved joints, improved the DJD. It also responded quite satisfactorily to oral nonsteroidal agents. The same basic program is used in treating inflammatory Rheumatoid Arthritis patients. What is obvious about osteoarthritis is that it does have a definite, clinical inflammatory component. The question is whether inflammation is secondary to trauma, or is one of the primary elements in osteoarthritis? Years of management have revealed that local injection of cortisone has definitely offered assistance degenerative joint disease management. The question of inflammation as an integral component is therefore more easily accepted.

Long-term experience and observation accentuate the disparity of placing causation of DJD with just the cartilage. Through close observation, during treatment of degenerative joint disease, conviction came that there was a mild inflammatory component in DJD formation: synovial inflammation as an important element in the process demanded to be heard. It's common to see middle-aged people with very mild inflammation - usually in the knees. Most often, it likely seems related to stress, trauma, or excess weight bearing, with the presence of synovial inflammation all to often being discounted while thinking of DJD's cause. A clinical question still needs to be addressed:

"Could the early synovial inflammation precede the ultimate embarrassment of the cartilage, resulting in premature and selective degeneration of the joint cartilage"? Such reasoning can account for the fact that it isn't unusual to see patients with severe DJD of the hips with knees spared or contrarily.

This without question is not a universally or generally accepted thesis, but one drawn by a conclusion of nearly half a century in observing and managing these various inflammatory and degenerative arthritic diseases.

An intermediary possibility is that it may actually have both origins. Mild inflammatory synovitis leads to damage of cartilage and more synovitis; while mild trauma ads cartilage damage, which may enhance synovitis, further damaging cartilage, "Osteoarthritis' circular Catch 22"[10]. Current therapeutic and biologic immunologic findings incorporated into the approach about synovial inflammation complements this thesis. Still, it will take a second-degree analysis of this concept to determine, if this idea shall prevail.

As a concluding thought to this wanton wading through perilous waters: DJD may be an inflammation of the synovium causing damage to cartilage, and damaged cartilage enhanced synovial inflammation - which involves one producing the other? That the basic cause is elusive is to be continuously remembered [Mr. Nobel knows]!

This hypothesis suggests that new biological treatment could conceptualize that by stopping the inflammation. That could mean joint replacement in the future may not be necessary[11].

VISUAL EVALUATION OF CARTILAGE

From conversations with a number of orthopedic surgeons fortified with 20 or more years of medical and surgical experience, I asked them to view from compiled concepts just what arthritis is from inside to outside. Previous brief dialogue showed how individually we medical and surgical practitioners carry unique ideas about the disease arthritis.

Visual, hands-on work of Orthopedists inspecting joints from within can provide us with important insights. Working with articular cartilage, surgeons have formulated ideas of what cartilage is and how it functions, responds, and what happen to it at various stages of activity. From the forces on cartilage within and outside the joint, more data can be discovered regarding this tissue.

Concurrently, rheumatologist are dealing with synovial tissue, touching, injecting, and attempting to control its proliferation. We are now understanding with greater specificity just what does occur within the joint with out ever-true visualization, Diagnostically and therapeutically, the pathologist is of no help but the orthopedic surgeon may be.

---

[10] *Catch-22* is a satirical, historical fiction novel by the American author Joseph Heller, first published in 1961

[11] *All these remarks about DJD as to its cause and the future management have undoubtedly been over emphasized and repeatedly over stated but the reasons are to punctuate these new ideas and concepts.*

What presently is known is that the biological activity in the synovium, and its synergism with the cartilage? This makes the orthopedic assessment and knowledge of cartilage extremely important. Comparison of the two tissues in this disease needs be undertaken for more complete knowledge as how damage occurs. The synergism that exists is a new subject for investigation.

A SUGGESTION FOR THE ORTHOPEDIC SURGEON

Within the synovium lies immunological activity. We now accept immune T-cells and B-cells are the source of the inflammatory disease. These T and B-cells biologically generate – for some inexplicable reason for some people - what we call *cytokines, which* include IL-1 and TNF-α - this latter one is the badest *baby: a* molecular substance that damages cartilage. Today, this is being clinically and systemically blocked with Enbrel, Humira, and Remicade.

This is the cutting edge of medical treatment of Inflammatory Arthritis. With that having proudly been said. Here is what one would like to see a collective group of orthopedic surgeons do with the next 50 or 100 surgically entered joints.

When in the joint visually and physically make note of both the synovium and cartilage;

Classify each into three categories. 1, 2, 3

Classifying the Synovia,

- Class 1 is nearly normal but slightly discolored, and with some perceptible swelling and inflammation;
- Class 2 has moderate proliferation, is hyperemic, and involved with vascularity that appears abnormal;
- Class 3 is Proliferated, and villous, and obviously severely inflamed.

Classifying Cartilages:

- Class 1 tissue is fairly normal with moderate damage;
- Class 2 tissue is abnormal overall, showing generalized abnormality.
- Class 3 tissue is very unhealthy with abnormal appearance, and is physically weak.

This would just be a brief classification with any other notation that the surgeon may deem to be appropriate. From this we will have gained appreciation and documentation of:

"Arthritis inside and out."

CHAPTER 7
EARLY ANTI-RHEUMATIC & ANTI-INFLAMMATORY DRUGS

As Rheumatology attracted great interest, the research into the development of drugs and pharmaceutical agents was spurred. This attention not only added to disease treatment, it provoked enquiry into causes of arthritic diseases. Medical schools and drug houses expanded their many research projects to assist diagnosis, treatment, with some attempting to find a cause and cure for the disease arthritis. The first true modern drug to treat and manage arthritis was aspirin.

The next great change came with the advent of steroids to treat Rheumatoid Arthritis. Treating RA with cortisone sparked interest in hormone metabolism. It also spurred investigation into the complications accompanying the use of cortisone. During this decade-long era, cortisone became the specialty of rheumatology. Cortisone being so widely used drastically changed our specialty. Because it happened fifty years ago, it was appropriate for it's being discussed earlier in this manuscript.

ASPIRIN, ITS HISTORY

It's taught that 2,500 years ago, Hippocrates, the ancestor of all doctors, treated pain in pregnant women, and fever with a bitter extract from the *willow bark*. This distillate contained salicylic acid, the origin of today's aspirin. Since then, salicylic acid, with its various compounds and mixtures, has been widely and successfully used in pain therapy, and in the treatment of arthritis. For decades, it was the unparalleled agent for treating the pain and inflammation of arthritis and all rheumatic diseases. That's why aspirin is the first therapeutic agent being discussed in this chapter.

Felix Hoffmann is credited with discovering aspirin – in as much as Hippocrates [550 BC] and Soranus [180 AD] left no truly expository journals for their descendents to offer the court in a 19th or 21st century lawsuit against Bayer. Hoffmann was born in Ludwigsburg, Germany in 1868 and was a dispensing chemist. After leaving school, he went to work in Geneva, Hamburg, and Neuveville. The work fascinated him to such an extent that he went to Munich to study pharmacy and chemistry. In 1891, he won his first degree while continuing to study chemistry, successfully completed his doctorate in 1903. He then worked at the Munich State

Laboratory before joining its then new and growing pharmaceutical industry.

On April 1, 1894, he began work at Farbenfabriken vorm Friedr. Bayer & Co. on the recommendation of one of its founders, Adolph von Bayer. He'd studied under him in Munich while working as a chemist. Shortly after that Felix Hoffmann discovered acetylsalicylic acid, which began being manufactured under the name *aspirin*. Soon, aspirin was known throughout the world. He, however, lived unrecognized until his death on February 8, 1946 in Switzerland, a not uncommon happenstance, who knows that Dennis Hunt invented the safety pin in 1880?

Over the past 100 years, aspirin has been used more than any other medication for the relief of pain. It was the first universally available pain reliever, and even today, it is used more than any other over the counter pain reliever and; it is used all over the world, though today it would never be approved by the FDA because it allows blood to run freely, and court dockets would be overwhelmed with megabuck lawsuits. Its effectiveness has, for years, been well established, but not until 1971 was it learned why aspirin was so effective in relieving pain and inflammation.

British pharmacologist, Sir John Vane, discovered the pain relief procedure: aspirin worked by inhibiting the body's production of a hormone-like substance called prostaglandin, an agent involved in the inflammatory process. Aspirin was also found to reduce the inflammation and swelling commonly associated with injuries, as well as from arthritis. Dr. Vane's research in this area received the Nobel Prize for Medicine in 1982.

DISCOVERING CORTISONE (COMPOUND E)

In 1948, Dr. Kendall isolated Compound E, later to be known as cortisone. His Mayo Clinic discovery introduced an entirely new direction for the specialty of Rheumatology. This one event in arthritis altered treatment to a greater extent than any other addition in the treatment of Rheumatoid Arthritis until modern times.

Dr. Philip Hench was a clinical investigator in rheumatology at the Mayo Clinic. He administered Dr. Kendall's Compound E to patients with severe Rheumatoid Arthritis. This test use can be considered the most dramatic major-therapeutic advancement ever made in treating arthritis. Once widely used, Compound E (Cortisone) revolutionized the treatment of Addison's disease, pituitary insufficiency, and Rheumatoid Arthritis. In 1950, Drs. Edward C. Kendall and Philip S. Hench, along with Tadeus Reichstein, a Swiss biochemist, shared the Nobel Prize in physiology and medicine for their work in isolating cortisone, and using it clinically to treat Rheumatoid Arthritis.

When Cortisone was initially used, RA was still marked - by the beliefs of the Osler period - as a hopelessly crippling and incurable disease. Many patients severely afflicted with Rheumatoid Arthritis never had any specific treatment to manage their ills, and were almost homebound by massively swollen, inflamed, painful joints; some being confined to a wheelchair. With the administration of Cortisone, which Dr. Hench prescribed as an injection, most patients felt a near-miraculous response.

One cannot recount enough times what this significant period meant to our specialty. During the 50's & 60's, a period of grand expectation came a revolutionary evolution in attitude about and approach to managing Rheumatoid Arthritis and rheumatic disease. It was generally felt that a cure for this devastating disease was in hand. Arthritis management, as well as the specialty of Rheumatology changed. Cortisone had entirely altered the morbidity of Rheumatoid Arthritis. The horizon lay clear.

CORTISONE FAILURE

Seven to ten years of steroid use resulted in a severe increase of cortisone side-effect complications. A variety of steroid compounds were tried to ascertain if side-effects and electrolyte imbalance could be eliminated, or at least controlled. Potassium loss and diabetic hyperglycemia were the major fears. None of these effects could be controlled; experience revealed they were steroids dose-related. During the 50's time of trouble, few other agents became available to truly alter the course of Rheumatoid Arthritis. RA remained an incurable, deforming, and crippling disease. There was only cortisone. Reconstructive surgery was still in its experimental stages when Cortisone's side effects began to prevail.

By the time it'd run its course, this drug went from grand expectations to fearsome anticipation. Expeditious efforts seeking alternative treatment methods were put on track. At cortisone's greatest utilization, all other standard agents had been shelved. Earlier drugs for treating RA were considered comparative failures, becoming historical footnotes. Those past therapeutic footnotes had to be reread so that earlier agents were again used in variety of ways.

In any case, experience with cortisone completely altered rheumatic diseases management regarding their diagnoses, and treatment. Following the decade of cortisone usage, it, and other steroids, whether oral or injected, was given lower respect while trying to understand how they brought relief.

The vacuum left by cortisone led to the beginning of joint aspiration as a diagnosis tool as well as a treatment of arthritis. Part of the Rheumatological training then was learning to perform an arthrocentesis, which was the aspiration and injection of arthritic joints. This procedure resulted in a unique skill that's now an integral part of rheumatology. Aspirating and injecting a joint is adequately performed with minimal discomfort, and can be done on most joints.

The era of belief in the all-powerful steroid having ended, the door opened for accepting a belief in anything else. Therapeutic programs were tried; clinical observations of the disease began learning more about RA during observations; RA appeared to improve during pregnancy – leading some to theorize that progesterone was a temporary aid. Inflammatory Arthritis diminished or disappeared during jaundice, typhoid, and many other infectious and inflammatory disease episodes. The first supposition was that these stressful states encouraged the body to produce its own cortisone, consequently temporarily abating the disease; time proved that this was not the case. An alternative guess was that an acute infectious problem causes the immune system to create antibody activity against this acute infection. The immune system being so diverted, their creating antibody aimed toward the arthritis was slowed. Following this, we tried to cure the disease with a large variety of agents affecting the immune system in attempts to stop, alter, or suppress Inflammatory Arthritis. Without specifying the details further, it is sufficient to state that all such trial-and-error efforts failed. RA was again being treated with aspirin.

A variety of other drugs and physical modalities were used. After being used decades earlier, gold injection was reborn for symptomatic relief. With little else available, it was believed that this treatment enhanced the possibility of altering and effecting Rheumatoid Arthritis remissions.

STEROID PROBLEMS REVISITED

Once started on oral steroids, the patient was totally incapable of stopping or eliminating the drug. This lifetime dependence is intolerable. Dependence and a host of complications, demanded that attention be directed to another treatment possibility had to come to the fore. But a decade or so before cortisone problems and complications became fully evident.

- Some of the first things seen were weight gain, occasionally from a voracious appetite.

- Facial hair developed.
- Thinning of the skin and stria (Stretch marks of the skin similar to those seen in pregnancy).
- Along with these was the typical 'Moon Face', round and red, as is seen in hypercortism or Cushing's disease. These finding were visual and evident.
- Peptic ulcer was probably the next complication seen from using steroids and occasionally mixing it with aspirin to diminish steroid dosage.
- Bleeding ulcers and GI hemorrhage was common. As usage continued, side-effects became problematic and more evident.
- Osteoporosis and compression fractures of the spine were seen with greater frequency.
- The eyes were involved when, cataracts developed from steroid use. If any drug was harmful to the eyes, it was cortisone and its derivatives; not Plaquenil, as was earlier described.
- There followed a metabolic change, with decreased potassium and increased fluid retention, salt retention, and hypertension.
- Along with these complications and problems, patients developed elevated blood glucose and, ultimately, diabetes.

Utilization of cortisone in treatment of RA and the complications as described encompassed a generation of disease management. Long-term steroid use was causing deaths, and rheumatology was dramatically changed forever by this period.

ALTERNATIVES TRIED AFTER CORTISONE.

In the 1950's, few physicians were being directed to the field of rheumatology. The total number of rheumatologists in the country was about one thousand. Since there were many unanswered questions in all phases of medicine, those attracted to treating arthritis aimed themselves mostly towards studying gout, infectious arthritis, and physical therapy.

On finding fewer practitioners, many patients sought comfort using whirlpool treatments. Many hospitals installed physical therapy departments, 'Hubbard' tanks, and other physical apparatus. The Hubbard tank is a huge, body-shaped stainless steel tub. The patient was placed on a canvas like stretcher, and immersed into it, to be fully bathed in warm, swirling water in a full body whirlpool. Many such devices had originally been developed to provide physiotherapy for poliomyelitis patients. This now gave birth to physiotherapy for RA rheumatoid patients. The Hubbard tank whirlpools, exercises, and wax treatment were reborn as 'new' technology treatment.

Melting sealing wax in a double boiler, dipping hands into the liquid, to form a warm glove was an ancient ritual. This was comforting but literally had no therapeutic effect. The effect of heat is locally soothing; ` it provides a feeling of comfort; causing the patient to believe it's therapeutically helpful. However, another consideration asks what heat does to a swollen joint? Well, it keeps the joint swollen and pained even though while using heat it is comforting. The early thought was that heat application increased circulation to the joint and that enhanced healing. In actuality, temporary comfort is all that was being offered. A more likely estimation is that it simply perpetuates the problem. The thought back then was that even in injury, heat was necessary to enhance circulation so as to hasten healing: counter-productive thinking! It took two generations to overcome this erroneous concept.

Many years later, an application of ice to swollen joints became acceptable. The use of ice in traumatic joints during athletic events demonstrated the method of local application to decrease swelling and, ultimately, a shortening of the disability.

Aggressively moving towards physiotherapeutic treatment after the cortisone period was a step backward. Dependence on such a modality received greater credence than it deserved. Experience with older modalities for a long time was shown to be a misuse. Because of the limited treatment available at that time, sending a patient to therapy was an acceptable alternative. There was not much else one could do, and this was a unique form of therapy. Sufferers would often return unhappy and hurting after being pushed through an exhausting pace by their enthusiastic therapist. Consequently, many patients no longer wanting to continue the treatment many would continue to endure the discomfort, believing that it was necessary for joint improvement. It took a re-schooled generation of therapists to begin handling arthritic patients for more gentile physiotherapy.

This form of treatment unfortunately is more helpful to the psyche, than hopeful for his physical state (his pneuma). While physiotherapy remains a cornerstone in the written description of most therapeutic writings on arthritis, the author feels its benefits are overstated enough to almost find a place in Chapter 4's follies list. Contrary to this belief every text on arthritis has large section devoted to physiotherapy.

While aged treatments were again being employed as an alternative to Cortisone, an almost frantic search was being pursued to find agents to manage and control Inflammatory Arthritis diseases. Numerous new and different agents were tried, employing trial-and-error. Their focus was on infection, or the immune system being out of sync. These considerations were all given credence for developing and in trying out new agents. On rare occasions, as previously noted, it was observed that, for individuals under stress from an infection, their RA improved. Based on this observation, antibiotics were used to treat Rheumatoid Arthritis and, after treating the specific infection, evaluation did indicate that patients' arthritis showed improvement. Acting on this observation, various antibiotics such as tetracycline, erythromycin, among others were used. An insidious infection was then considered a possible cause of RA, so all infections needed to be expunged from the body. This new concept, however, had once been prevalent; then, it resulted in full-mouth extraction of teeth to remove what was considered a focus of infection, illustrating how far back infection was considered as a cause of RA.

Rheumatoid Arthritis is associated with many systemic problems, one of which is colitis or irritable colon. In a small number of patients with the disease, the association of flare-ups sometimes coincides with an increase in bowel symptoms. As a result, Azulfidine (combination of sulfa pyridine and 5-aminosalicylic acid) was specifically manufactured for bowel symptom treatment. It was a weak, poorly absorbed sulfa compound mixed with salicylates. The idea was to change the bacterial flora in the GI tract. By doing this, it was assumed that there would be less challenge to the immune system.

In the inflamed mucous membranes of the bowel, a larger than normal amount of bacteria could challenge the immune system via a transient bacterial stimulation of the patient's altered bowel activity. Influx of bacteria into the circulation stimulates antibody formation to kill bacteria. They also act to stimulate the RA patient's body to produce antibodies, which then flare-up his arthritis. By changing the bacteria content of the bowel, one could have a therapeutic effect on a possible stimulus of the arthritic activity in some patients. Consequently, many patients with RA received, and are receiving, Azulfidine as a disease-modifying agent. Unfortunately, the conceptual idea is measurably effective in only 10 or 15% of RA patients concomitantly having bowel symptoms.

For years, it also had been taught that most RA cases could be traced to a severe emotional crisis. Students were taught to seek this in their history taking. It was even suggested a cause affecting acute flare-ups of arthritis. Many such patients received psychiatric treatment in order to arrest the disease. However, any chronic illness is understandably associated with some depression; depression is no more than a supportive result – an effect, not a cause

GOLD THERAPY GETS BORN AGAIN

Gold had been used for centuries to treat arthritis, as it was for many other diseases such as tuberculosis. After cortisone, there was nothing innovative or new to treat RA. By the beginning of the last half of the last century, it became the real 'Gold Standard' for treatment. It was given in frequent, increasing doses until a maintenance dose and interval was determined. Initially the intramuscularly dose received was ten mgm [that's science-speak for milligrams]. This was increased weekly to twenty mgm, thirty, forty, and ultimately fifty mgm every two weeks. Patients usually received injections of this amount every two weeks until they had a cumulative dose of 500 mgm. A full and therapeutic dose was a cumulative dose of one gram. The usual dose progressed to fifty mgm a month. One hoped to see a demonstrable effect from 500 mgm. The optimum was a remission at a gram or more. During this period, physicians and patients alike generally felt that there was a clinical response and the disease was under better control. Gold became a standard and favorite treatment for Rheumatoid Arthritis.

Time and greater experience resulted in a variation of both dosage, and combining gold with other drugs. Enthusiast physicians and patients were convinced that gold was a helpful agent in altering the disease. It was felt that gold potentially could bring remission. For a generation, gold was the treatment of choice. A patient with Rheumatoid Arthritis who hadn't had a clinical trial of treatment with gold felt he hadn't been managed properly. Most rheumatologists accepted gold's promising premise. Gold had moved from a long-ago feared, rather radical, somewhat dangerous technique into a commonplace treatment.

In its early history, gold had developed a very bad reputation among patients and the general population who considered it very dangerous. Even many of those with severe disease, were reluctant to try gold injections. Time demonstrated that it was quite safe when closely monitored. One patient received cumulative doses of gold weighing 20,000 mgm - almost an ounce of gold - in one full course of treatment. Some individuals actually received doses as high as 100 mgm of gold twice a month for years. Gold therapy became standard for decades and, as was noted, some apparent remissions occurred. Little was known of the action of gold other than its clinical observations. Use of gold varied among rheumatologists; doses were administered differently. It stood alone in this method of managing the disease. Some cynical consideration held that its therapeutic effect was mainly psychological. More cynical was the 'saw' that physicians administering it used it only to en-golden their revenue.

GOLD AND MORE GOLD

Gold does work, and it did affect the disease. Its major drawback is that its positive effect wasn't universal, and years of administering it resulted in a paucity of actual remissions, and few RA modifications. Originally, it was used for severe disease, but in time, almost all patients with Rheumatoid Arthritis of any sort were being offered the drug as a treatment. Later studies seemed to indicate the mode of action of gold was its effective inhibition of monocytes suppressing the immune system.

Primary manuscripts and texts on rheumatology – e.g. ascent as Hollander and McCarty's Eighth Edition of *Arthritis* [chapter 29]; and our esteemed rheumatologists: Richard Fryberg, Morris Ziff, and John Baum - stated in their discourse on gold:

"The manner in which gold works is unknown."

This represented a classic example of how agents began their use in treating Rheumatoid Arthritis. It was primarily by trial that gold, through multiple treatment trials, would or would not prove to be effective. Gold was first used in treating tuberculosis where it was found to inhibit growth of TB bacilli. Ziff later produced studies that suggested gold inhibited enzyme transfer in macrophages. Inhibiting Macrophage enzyme transfer was then considered gold's mode of action because those enzymes caused inflammation. This suggested activity only materialized many years after decades of using gold therapeutically as an effective agent in treating RA.

One cannot overstate the magnitude of the use of gold as the major treatment of Rheumatoid Arthritis during this period. However, much was happening contemporaneously. The major question was, what was the effect of each agent utilized on an individual, or to or her immune system? Another area of concern was how was this, or any other program, affecting the quality of life of the particular RA patient. Many rheumatologists, after years of treating this disease and those patients living daily with RA, wondered if indeed this drug was effective"

DISEASE MODIFYING DRUGS

Constant search began again for agents (such as Cupramine, Cyclophosphamide, and Azathioprine which are to be mentioned below) that would not only decrease inflammation but also modify the course of Rheumatoid Arthritis. The investigation was for agents to attack the considered cause within the immune system. These were termed disease modifying and remitting drugs, or DMARD's. During this developmental period, there was a fixation of there being a positive rheumatoid factor in the blood. It was felt that the severity of the disease was related to a Rheumatoid Factor (RF) protein and to its level. To a minor extent, this was true, but not universally true. As a result, Penacillamine (Cupramine), a chelating agent, was found able to lower that RF by binding this immunoglobulin and enhancing its excretion. This was then used liberally; it had minimal effect used alone or in combination. Combinations of these DMARD's were then frequently used. After years of dispensing Penacillamine this was eliminated as a useful anti-rheumatic agent.

The next drug varieties to be employed were immunosuppressant. They were tried and used frequently in attempts to alter and control RA and other inflammatory diseases. These categories of drugs were known as immunosuppressant drugs. Many had found past use in treating various forms of cancer. Cytoxan (Cyclophosphamide) was a drug used for a number of years in cancer management. Its use became popular in an attempt to poison immune T and B-cells, involved in the activity of the disease. This and other drugs were agents used in chemotherapy for breast cancer. It also was noted that, while on chemotherapy, RA activity diminished. These women were frequently on Prednisone (steroid) Cytoxan and another suppressant agent (three drugs.) As a result, Cytoxan was utilized to treat Rheumatoid Arthritis and other rheumatic diseases. Its use was mostly another desperate attempt to find a replacement for cortisone. For some years, it was used but never succeeded as a disease-managing agency. Another such agent used, but to a lesser degree, was Imuran, or Azathioprine. This also was an attempt to find a useful immunosuppressant agent. These agents brought some theoretical approach to attacking the disease but were far from being adequate or practical.

PLAQUENIL

Generically speaking, proliferations of drugs to treat arthritis were being produced, but all were quite mild and not very effective. The desperation in treating severe Rheumatoid Arthritis resulted in drugs being added to drugs in various combinations. Concern then developed regarding polypharmacy and the therapeutic use of multiple chemicals. What developed was an increased number of agents considered to have a remitting, or disease-modifying, effect.

For a time, our dicta were 'go slow' and 'build on' one's therapeutic approach. The drug regime that was advocated by teaching programs was a diagrammed pyramid. On the bottom was aspirin. Climbing up to the pyramid's next level was Plaquenil, an antimalarial drug now expected to be useful in modifying the disease. This antimalarial was ascertained to be effective for various patients in controlling their arthritis. As would be expected, as potential agents numerically increased, the number of levels increased with the most potent agent supposed to rest atop the therapeutic pyramid. This form of categorizing therapeutic agents grew impractical.

Plaquenil (Hydroxychloroquine sulfate) was found to be modestly effective in modifying the rheumatic diseases with prolonged use. With ease of administration, 200 to 400 mgm of Plaquenil was taken orally on a daily basis. It was used almost routinely in Rheumatoid Arthritis and connective tissue diseases. As with most drugs used, its entrance into the armamentarium was accidental. Widespread use of Chloroquin (Plaquenil is a durative) occurred in the military for malaria; that led to an observation on its benefit for RA patients. Side-effects of Plaquenil are minimal, however there are instances of GI disturbance and occasionally a rash. Its effectiveness is quite limited and used primarily for mild cases.

Years later, it was learned that combinations of agents were more effective and Plaquenil was one of the drugs frequently used in this manner. Plaquenil has been used in combination with anti-inflammatory agents and later, even in combination with gold and many other anti-rheumatic drugs. The old, progressive pyramid concept became passé. The increased number of available agents was not very effective for a severely aggressive Rheumatoid Arthritis. Sometimes RA management appeared to be fighting like an insurgent war. RA's internal enemy has never been successively well identified, striking at unanticipated times in unsuspected places. Repulsing each attack of the disguised adversary is like putting down another surprising uprising. This insurgent warfare is almost constant, and needs to be approached aggressively. One dare never become complacent or quit.

Whenever the use of a new agent was spread widely, it became common to look for adverse effects and problems. Frequently in medicine, side-effects are reported, sometimes overstated, and their non-existence or exaggeration is difficult to refute.

In the late fifties the Cleveland Clinic had an article claiming that one of the serious side-effects of long-standing use of Plaquenil was retinal damage. It described the occurrence of retinal pigmentation from the prolonged use of Plaquenil with ultimate damage to the eyes with possibly impaired vision. Consequently, there have been millions and millions of special opthamological eye examinations and negligible such findings

CHAPTER 8
REPLACING STEROID TREATMENT
NONSTEROIDAL ANTI-INFLAMMATORY AGENTS (NSAID's)

*I*n the 1970's, the growth, development, management, and treatment of arthritis was discovering modalities that would control the disease, which were void of the complications of steroids, and without any new problems.

Educational institute purists suggested that treatment should, first of all, be focused on maximized doses of aspirin; after all, Cortisone was heavily used systemically until its problems appeared and aspirin had a millennial-long almost placebo-like history. Some felt that salicylization meant using high doses of aspirin to near toxicity. Coated aspirin usually was the drug of choice to achieve this state. Twelve to sixteen coated aspirins were suggested as a daily dosing. After years of devastating steroids, rheumatological educational circles concluded that aspirin, in general, was adequate to safely manage the inflammatory process. It didn't take long to learn that such thinking was unrealistic.

Patients didn't receive the relief desired, and they just couldn't tolerate it for long periods: GI distress was rampant; decreased hearing was another major problem as well as allergic reactions. With cortisone considered forbidden fruit, rheumatologists had to relearn ways of management without that most useful agent. Treatment turned towards following a process of seeking out an acceptable way to replace cortisone, while still controlling the disease, as has Cortisone. Fear had stricken the management program that once had considered it was holding the Cure-of-cures. During its evolution in treating Rheumatoid Arthritis and other arthritic conditions, Rheumatology had repeatedly progressed through its share of shock episodes.

Physician organizations with pharmaceutical companies rallied by coming up with what they termed NSAID's - non-steroidal anti-inflammatory drugs. These were the first new compounds used to treat Inflammatory Arthritis. All arrived with great expectations. Although helpful, they never fulfilled all that was promised. The grand expectation was that these drugs would relieve inflammation as well as steroids. For a dozen years, a new agent was annually released by a variety of drug companies. Each one promised to outperform the earlier one. It became such a heated pharmaceutical area that every drug company had to have an NSAID. The market for an effective anti-inflammatory medication was desperately large.

Steroid replacement was needed. It clearly was necessary for some agent or agents to suppress the disease; the Plaquenil used earlier now became one of the drugs most prescribed to modify rheumatoid disease. One by one, agents and items were considered and tried: none were new. Even so, almost every old treatment was again prescribed in various dosages and combinations. The teaching was to *go slow* and add one agent at a time to *build on.* This therapeutic pyramid approach stepped through: Aspirin; Plaquenil; Cupramine; and various DMARD's like: Sulfasalazine, a sulfa anti-inflammatory salicylates; Oral gold; Aranafin; Cytoxan; and Imuran. Darvocet (propoxaphine), among many other pain drugs ancillary to the pyramid, were added to the prescription pads of desperate rheumatologists. Some of these have been mentioned in the previous chapter, with many of them in definitive detail.

Now it's time to examine more closely those drugs specifically under development during the treatment slowdown in the post-cortisone era.

INTRODUCTION OF NSAID's

During the 1970s there was at least a new NSAID each year, with each proposing to deliver more and greater benefits. These agents had analgesic, anti-inflammatory, antipyretic and antiplatelet properties. The action of these agents was to inhibit COX enzymes to decrease prostaglandin production. The two families were the earlier traditional COX-1, and the more newly developed COX-2. These sets differ in their individual function and in the tissue through which they are distributed. The COX-1 (NSAID's) affected prostaglandin and prostacyclins of the stomach, which maintain the stomach's mucosal integrity. The COX-1 decreased prostaglandin, which accounted for those agents harming the GI tract. They also affect vaso-regularity, which accounts for their effect on the kidney and its circulation.

The COX-2 drugs were more recently introduced and their varied effects have garnered wider interest since their anti-inflammatory effect is much greater. They are reported to effect ovulation, have little platelet effect, and cause less bleeding. There's generally less GI erosions and a lowered colonic effect. Initial descriptions claimed they might have less effect on kidney and edema. Increased use of the COX-2 drugs however proved its contrary: these drugs can cause excessive fluid retention resulting in increased blood pressure, which is exaggerated in those who primarily suffer from hypertension. Consequently, this major negativity has resulted in two such agents being withdrawn. Major litigation continues as this easily understood and documented clinical event seeks resolution.

Each new nonsteroidal agent attempted to offer its greater anti-inflammatory advantage with its fewer side-effects. Since their basic chemistries were only slightly different, all NSAID's behaved similarly. All were directed towards blocking the active inflammation complex. The more potent the NSAID, the greater it disturbed stomach-mucosa - that almost became a rule. Much of the time an NSAID had a direct topical effect: the stomach lining burned due to increased acid production. Along with this, the effect on prostaglandin decreased its protective mucin content, further embarrassing stomach linings. This had been discovered only after years of greater experience with these drugs.

An early new drug added to the list of NSAID's was Ansaid. It was similar to Motrin, a product of the same company, Upjohn, who marketed it as an improvement to Motrin. It was far superior in decreasing inflammation, but extremely irritating to the upper GI tract – do we detect a correlation? Very few patients were able to tolerate Ansaid. This appropriately named drug remained a useful agent but only for a short time. Another interesting agent was the first only once-a-day dosage, Feldene; it initially provided a major advantage over other available NSAID's with need to be taken more often. It, moreover, was quite a potent anti-inflammatory drug. Unfortunately, after increased usage, it was found to suddenly cause severe gastric hemorrhaging. The acute hemorrhage came about with almost no symptoms to alert the individual that he was bleeding. This anti-inflammation analgesic apparently eliminated pain, making distress in an inflamed stomach and/or ulcer, hemorrhaging unnoticeable: this terrible hazard was occurring suddenly and silently. The circumstance of such drug activity was more than happenstance; the manufacturer never actually accepted this as fact. It occurred so frequently that the drug eventually was only used in selective patients who had been started on it and, thankfully, tolerated it without a GI problem. For those that tolerated Feldene, it was an exceptionally helpful agent, but their number was small.

With early acceptance for the use of Feldene, Lilly quickly released a drug called Oraflex, another once-a-day NSAID. At the same time, Lilly sent 'news releases' to the media - a not accepted procedure at that time. With the release of Oraflex the manufacturer claimed possible curative results for RA sufferers. The resultant clamor for it was astounding! The demand from the public for this agent deluged practicing physicians. Sufferers insisted on trying the drug, causing willing doctors to take personal responsibility for possible problems. Oraflex was selling for about one dollar per capsule. It became almost an impossible task to ward off insistent patients wanting to abandon their present medication - so eager were they to give Oraflex a one month try. After one month, a great number of individuals were on Oraflex. It was quite an effective anti-inflammatory agent. Public attempts were made to persuade the drug company to cease its aggressive advertising campaign. But it had paid physicians to make these over-enthusiastic claims, so they persisted in defending its campaign. With all the publicity Lilly created, in England it was discovered within a month, there had been a few never disclosed deaths in early clinical trials.

The backlash against the company was enormous. Oraflex was removed from the market, never to be used again. Some believed that the entire episode was a mistake, and that Oraflex probably was neither as effective as announced, nor as harmful as reported. It, indeed, may have been superior to the drug it was challenging. Oraflex's true worth was never determined.

PROLIFERATION OF NSAID's AVAILABLE

The below list illustrates the large number of NSAID's that had become available. They are represented in the order they became available. Not listed are Butazolidine or Indocin, which were years earlier and not generally categorized with NSAID's, but are non-steroidal as is aspirin also not listed. Much of the listing is categorical according to era it was released.

- Motrin, 400 mgm (Ibuprofen); its chemical name is 2,4-isobutylphenylpropionic acid.
- Naprosyn, 250 mgm. Naproxen and naproxen sodium are (S)-6-methoxy- (alpha)-methyl-2-naphthaleneacetic acid
- Tolectin, 400 mgm. Chemically Sodium 1 methyl-5- (4-methylbenzoyl)-1H-pyrrole-2-acetate dihydrate
- Nalfon, 200 mgm. (Fenopenfen calcium) Benzeneacetic acid, (alpha)-methyl-3-phenoxy-
- Ansaid,100-mgm.(Flurbiprofen)(+)-2-(2-fluoro-4 biphenylyl) propionic
- Dolobid, 250 mgm. (Meclofenamic Acid)
- Clinoril, 200 mgm. (Sulindac) (Z)-5-fuloro-2 methyl 1-1 (p-methylsulfinyl phenyl)methylene)-1H-indene-3 acetic acid
- Lodine, 200 mgm. (Etodolac) 1,8-diethyl-1,3,4,9-tetrahydropyrano-(3,4-b)indole-1-acetic acid
- Feldene, 20 mgm. (Piroxicam) 4-hydroxyl-2-methyl-N-2-pyridinyl-2H-1,2,-benzothiazine-3-carboxamide 1.1-dioxide

- <u>Orival</u>, 25 mgm. (ketoprophin)
- <u>Voltarin</u>, 50 mgm. (Diclophenac)
- <u>Catiflam</u>, 50 mgm.(diclofenac potassium)
- <u>Relafin</u>, 500 mgm. (Nabumetone)
- <u>Orudis</u>, 25 mgm. (Ketoprophin)
- <u>Toradol</u>, 10 mgm.(ketorolac tromethamine)
- <u>Ponstil</u>, 250 mgm. (Meclofenamate)
- <u>Daypro</u>, 600 mgm. (Oxaprozin)
- <u>Arthrotec</u>, 75 mgm. (Diclophenac and Cytoxina
- <u>Celebrex</u>, 100 mgm. (celecoxib)
- <u>Vioxx</u>, 12.5 mgm. (rofecoxib)
- <u>Mobic</u>, 7.5 mgm. (Meloxicam)
- <u>Bextra</u>, 20 mgm. (valdecoxib)

It generally takes some two years to fully evaluate the effectiveness of such drugs, and to discover if they have a lasting therapeutic effect. It took this long to determine if a promising NSAID was efficacious and really does have promise. However, various companies never allowed for full evaluation of each drug, how well it works, or check out its true toxicity. Since the Oraflex debacle, pharmaceutical companies have become more discreet – sometimes obstinately so.

Minor problems have occurred with all NSAID's. They, however, were very helpful in managing arthritis: they were all analgesic and mildly anti-inflammatory, but none altered the course of the disease as marketers proclaimed in their news releases. The usual claim was, 'studies showed decreases in bone erosion'. Practically speaking, findings regarding the healing of erosion failed, to prove such a claim, even after years of use, but widespread use of NSAID's continued. Today, they are commonly used, in smaller doses, and are as safe as aspirin when used for moderate symptom relief. From the powerful anti-rheumatic agents that offered cures and - despite great fear of toxicity - NSAID agents ultimately became over-the-counter pharmaceuticals.

As described, the major side-effect materializing from NSAID's was on the stomach lining and the GI tract because they block the production of prostaglandin. NSAID gastropathy was the label given to this side-effect. Gastropathy can occur with small or short-course treatment, or can be cumulative occurring months or years later. The most serious problem is bleeding; it can occur from the severe inflammation, or from ulceration with all its symptoms and complications. It became an NSAID treatment predicament. The longer the use of these agents, and the larger the dose, the more assuredly will there be a GI tract problem. As a result, there was much duplication and agent-redundancies. Over the years, arthritis drugs have created a unique relationship between the pharmaceutical industry and rheumatology. The continual stream of NSAID's released created a drug era similar to the cortisone period. Because of the problems with Oraflex and Lilly - as mentioned earlier - this indelibly led rheumatologists into skepticism.

NONSTEROIDAL ANTI-INFLAMMATORY DRUGS
AND MANAGING GI DISTRESS

Part of the discussion of NSAID's must include the GI problems that tend to result. Because this represents the activity of secondary side-effect of these drugs, more discussion is to follow in order to further clarity how wide use resulted, along with an over-the-counter availability for these drugs.

Each company making these drugs came up with its own better and more powerful agent. In the long run, the most interesting thing that developed was that there was a fair amount of individual tolerance and efficacy for these drugs. In general, all acted the same; all had the same adverse effects. The most evident finding was that the more potent an anti-inflammatory, the greater the undesirable chance of an adverse GI effect. Universally, they'd produce gastric irritation, ulcers, and potential bleeding. NSAID's that were not as problematic were also not very effective in controlling pain and inflammation. These agents were used in great quantities over the years, often combining with many other drugs. Basically, these substitutes never replaced steroids.

The latest method of NSAID utilization is to instruct the patient to use them only on demand according to the symptoms and necessity. Past thinking had been to provide a constant dose in order to achieve a blood level to suppress the inflammation and its symptoms. Unfortunately, this generally produced GI problems. This modern approach allows for better and longer effectiveness and compliance of these agents.

Over the years, the most onerous and least well handled and monitored effect is still GI bleeding. Platelet coating inhibiting coagulation effects bleeding. This is a hazard for the elderly and is being described by some practitioners, as possibly a fatal complication. To this date, over-the-counter NSAID's are labeled to be 'a severe health hazard for the elderly'. Anyone, while on these drugs, should be closely monitored for GI bleeding. This doesn't suggest overuse of gastroscopy, colonoscopy, or GI x-rays - even frequent stool analyses for occult blood are not necessary. If done routinely, they can complicate the picture. By far, the most important test is monitoring the hematocrit and hemoglobin. At the first sign of a drop in the blood count, blood loss needs to be immediately confirmed. Most of the time, the drop in blood count is subtle: it occurs very slowly, causing anemia. Frequently, there was no history of noticeable blood loss or black stools.

As once mentioned, this highly-suspicious author has, over his last thirty-five years, observed about three GI cancers and other lesions annually - that amounts to a hundred cases. The vast majority are early lesions that may not have been symptomatic over the previous years: almost all the patients reported a cure. One could conclude that it was the enhancement of the bleeding tendency that caused these occult lesions to bleed and become detected. Might this consequence of a side-effect have produced a good result? In this regard, these nonsteroidal drugs are actually life saving if there is close observation for bleeding and a high index of suspicion. This unique observation is not reported as a positive benefit versus a potentially serious problem from these drugs.

COX-2 NONSTEROIDALS

With this agent from the later part of the twentieth century, we have the first modern introduction of a new anti-rheumatic pharmaceutical agent. Almost a quarter of a century had passed before the industry produced a new anti-rheumatic agent. In that period, clinical use, or medical and therapeutic fads and fripperies, provided all that was new in so-called drugs and agents.

Celebrex, when released, was the first new anti-rheumatic drug of any kind since we began using Methotrexate. This category of anti-inflammatory was not a great advancement in our drug armory aimed at treating arthritis, but it possessed a safety factor. Celebrex, a nonsteroidal anti-inflammatory drug, exhibits anti-inflammatory, analgesic, and antipyretic activities in animal models. Celebrex' mechanism of action is believed to be via inhibition of prostaglandin synthesis, primarily by inhibition of cyclooxygenase-2 (COX-2). Another step had just been taken to chemically proceed closer to the inflammation mechanism and to block its response. An ultimate agent would inhibit it from happening altogether. Each chemical step is moving us closer to attacking – and perhaps solving - the destructive problem of inflammation in joints.

The major effect of Celebrex was directed at treating inflammatory symptoms. As had all other nonsteroidal drugs, it possessed an ability to perform, as it professed, with a far lower deleterious effect on the gastrointestinal tract. Although, when this drug was released, the company was very successful in its sales marketing, Celebrex and other Cox-2 drugs were unable to alter the course of Rheumatoid Arthritis. It was another in a long line of agents to manage the inflammatory state that couldn't modify or suppress the disease; it was easier on the GI tract.

Vioxx was the next new nonsteroidal anti-inflammatory drug to exhibit anti-inflammatory, analgesic, and antipyretic activities in animal models. It is believed to inhibit prostaglandin synthesis via inhibition of cyclooxygenase-2 (COX-2). At therapeutic concentrations in humans, Vioxx doesn't inhibit the cyclooxygenase-1 (COX-1) isoenzyme. That's similar to Celebrex; its promotion campaign was also similar. Vioxx was another agent of the same chemical type to become available. Because all these agents have patient specificity, additional drugs are always acceptable.

Its drug insert states: *"Food had no significant effect on either the peak plasma concentration (C max) or extent of absorption (AUC) of rofecoxib when VIOXX tablets were taken with a high fat meal. The time to peak plasma concentration (T max), however, was delayed by 1 to 2 hours. The food effect on the suspension formulation has not been studied. VIOXX tablets can be administered without regard to timing of meals."*

It's been noted and recorded that excess fluid retention is a by-product from the use of this anti-inflammatory, but this is common in all such agents. Management can be achieved by monitoring and restricting of fluid intake. The greatest problem isn't being aware of the property of fluid retention. This frequently is coupled with the *'old wives tale'* that one must drink at least eight glasses of water each day, or the forcing of a large amount of liquid with the impression that it has some therapeutic effect of washing out whatever that's bad or harmful.

Vioxx, and other drugs, enhancing the body's property of fluid retention can cause expanded blood volume, hypertension, and all the existing consequences that may result. One mustn't lose sight of the fact that the initial treatment of hypertension is the administration of a diuretic. Fluid restriction can have the same effect on hypertension and the need for a diuretic or fluid restriction. Therefore, when using these drugs, an individual, at risk for such an outcome, needs to be constantly aware of fluid retention.

In marketing Vioxx, the aforementioned potential eventualities were never part of the informative parcel promoted by its manufacturer. Consequently this very effective - and possible the best of the nonsteroidals - has been removed by the manufacturer because of its association with patients who died of heart disease.

Mobic was the latest new NSAID to arrive. In 2000, a large German company [Boehringer Ingelheim Pharmaceuticals] released it to our country. In competing with the new Cox-2 drugs, its major claim was that it also was structured to be less damaging to the stomach and GI tract than earlier once-a-day NSAID's. It's been well received. However, it takes years to determine any NSAID's lasting value and its ability to sustain its use as an agent worthy to manage arthritis.

CHAPTER 9
JOINT ASPIRATION AND INJECTION

Physicians on employing joint aspiration as a diagnostic technique, another treatment modality came into existence.

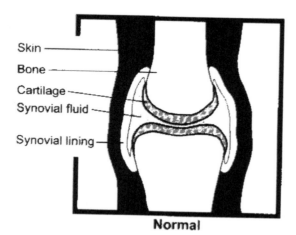

Normal

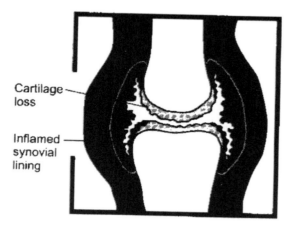

Arthritis.

𝐽 oint fluid first interested investigators when they began checking for uric acid crystals; this was to determine if gout was the joint's problem, or to determine if infection was present. Aspiration became quite common.

- To assess what was going on in hot swollen joints;
- To search for crystalline arthritis as was found in gout;
- To seek an infection causing the severity of inflammation.
- To determine specific finding characteristics of the joint fluid in Rheumatoid

Much was made of the color and character of the joint fluid in RA, be it clear, cloudy, and/or viscous. Also reported were the number and quantity of cells, and the viscosity of the fluid. The more inflamed, the less viscous was an assumption because inflammation decreased the mucin content of joint fluid. Rheumatoid factor was also measured in hope it might become a severity predictor for RA. As joint aspiration became more prevalent, it evolved into the diagnostic tool of Rheumatology. None of these features in the joint fluid of Rheumatoid or other arthritis bore any predictable therapeutic, or morbidity information, unless infection was present.

The major problems that *did* result in the past included the introduction of bacteria into the joint by employing bacteria-transferring non-disposable syringes and needles until disposable-syringes and needles were available. Another problem was the acute flare-up that occurred shortly after an injection of the hydrocortisone. Follow-up aspiration was preformed to be certain that infection hadn't occurred. It was later determined that flare-up was a direct-result from crystals of hydrocortisone being injected. This created a situation similar to the action of uric acid crystals found in gout sufferers. Based on this, drug companies sought to manufacture drugs having different crystalline compositions for injectable cortisone agents. It was noted that aqueous cortisone was rapidly absorbed and did have a systemic effect also, just as an intramuscular or intravenous injection of a steroid, but it was short lived and remained associated with all the side-effects of oral cortisone.

Here seems an appropriate place to inject the tale of why injection of cortisone into inflamed joints was so slow in coming: an orthopedic research lab, in order to prove Cortisone's danger, injected large amounts of it into the knee joints of dogs and actively exercised them. After carefully observation for weeks, the dogs were sacrificed and found to have severely damaged cartilage. This study - and much hearsay - promulgated negative attitudes regarding joint injection with cortisone and like agents: it was an attitude persisting for years. It was later demonstrated that the doses injected were over 100 times more concentrated than used in an adult human. It's taken generations to counter this report; even today, some residual hesitation still exists.

Universal thinking and treatment about and with medicine was still in its infancy at this time. Neither drug companies would advertise, nor could physicians. The American Medical Association was still a powerful and well-respected repository for medical information and credibility. Older physicians ran the AMA, and it took years and sometimes generations for a bad idea to change, or for a new drugs and procedures to be accepted. Advances in medicine and disease control came about via individual management patterns. Change took years even under the influence of reports from respected physicians, clinics, or medical schools.

As a consequence, injecting inflamed joints with steroid products was used for decades while never being recognized as a foundation stone for treating with Rheumatoid Arthritis patients. Centers of learning, during this period, continued to hold it in disrepute, while physicians treating active patients used it more and more. Acceptance of a new idea often becomes a lengthy process.

Its use started creeping into rheumatology books and periodicals, but the national arthritis organizations took decades before allowing a formal paper to be presented on the topic of injecting cortisones into local joints. Even today, the use and technique is modestly taught in medical schools. With oral cortisone in disrepute, local injections were finding a place for control and management of arthritis. There was little doubt as to the efficacy or effect of intra-articular corticosteroids on Rheumatoid Arthritis. The questions to be answered were, which were the best agents, and what harm vs. benefit would be derived. In time, all these questions were answered. When these agents are injected, there's no question that there is systemic absorption. How much and how long depended on the characteristics of the crystals used. If too much was given, and too often, the same effect came into play as in oral agents, and the patient could become 'Cushioned'. Decades of use produced the following conclusions,

- Introduction of infection was nearly nonexistent when the area was cleaned with Betadine (povadine-iodine 10%) and disposable syringes and needles were used.
- Post injection flare from the injected crystals was minimal, 1-5% when DepoMedrol (methylprednisolone acetate), or Aristocort (Triamcinalone actinide) were used.
- Damage to the joint didn't occur from the steroid itself.
- If injections are given at an interval of every two months at 40 mgm doses, the duration of use can be almost indefinite.
- Some patients can have a hormonal flush following an injection.
- It is the single most effective way to control an acute inflamed and swollen joint.
- It is the safest way to reduce acute pain and swelling of an isolated joint.
- On occasion, multiple joints can be injected.
- Injections, too often and too close together, can lose effectiveness, just as oral steroids did in the past.
- It is nearly impossible to manage and treat Rheumatoid Arthritis, over long periods, without this modality.
- It is effective in Degenerative Joint Disease, thereby assessing the inflammatory nature of this disease.
- To be most effective, a joint that has any appreciable amount of fluid (effusion), this excess fluid should be removed at the same time to prevent the dilution of the steroid.
- It has even been used in acute gouty joints.

- The declaration of absolute contraindication in an infected joint is not supported by vast clinical experience.

This aspiration technique is the safest and surest way of locally treating acute pain, inflammation, and supplementing other concurrent systemic treatment for an acutely inflamed joint. Over the decades, intra-articular injection of steroid preparations has developed into a much-used procedure but still some seem to harbor feelings of coercion. The past generation had added no new agents, information, hazards, or concerns to the use of joint injections of corticosteroids.

A final note of import is that when a steroid injection into a joint does not have measurable beneficial effect, the conclusion is inflammation must be minimal and the majority of the pain is most likely mechanical.

CHAPTER 10
THE ERA OF METHOTREXATE

In attempting to master the disease upon the disuse of steroids, many agents, and procedures were tried.

*T*reatment of RA had taken a sharp turn away from steroids-only into designing a management plan. Even exchange transfusions were attempted. Exchange transfusions of blood were done mostly at the Cleveland Clinic. Their hoped-for-expectation was that, by removing active abnormal elements of Rheumatoid Arthritis from their blood, RA conditions would be improved.

Selection, from a catalog of available agents, about which drug to be utilized was greatly influenced by what was the newest anti-inflammatory anti-rheumatic agent. Most often, it was a new nonsteroidal agent. One had to sort through an assemblage of agents, as well as the 'spin' attached to them. Ultimately, it was the physician who determined and selected the best agent that could be tolerated by the patient as well as being most effective in controlling inflammation: an NSAID was usually picked.

Pain control was always the major consideration, along with safe and tolerable not far behind, Codeine and/or Darvocet often filled the bill. What was needed for the disease management was an agent designed to suppress or modify RA. Gold injections or possibly one of the DMARD's (disease-modifiers) such as Plaquenil, Cupramine, Azulfidine (combination of sulfapyridine and 5-aminosalicylic acid), Cytoxan, or Imuran were used. Complementing this would be an occasional injection of a local acting steroid, such as Aristacort or DepoMedrol into the joint. This management program used a conglomeration of drugs. Each set was planned on understanding the patient, and his disease. The set was customized to meet tolerability, compliance, and best efficacy standards, so as not to bring about distress or side-effects.

The time for Methotrexate began slowly and subtly[11]. This agent had been available for years and was originally used to treat leukemia in children. Dermatologists used it to treat a small numbers of patients with severe psoriasis, using much larger doses. Many psoriasis patients also had arthritis. It was noted that Methotrexate appeared to have a therapeutic

---

[11] This represents the classic example of the off label use of a drug (Methotrexate) and especially in treating arthritis where this has usually been the norm.

effect on Rheumatoid Arthritis. Methotrexate, at that time, had acquired a bad safety reputation due to reports of liver toxicity with severe liver damage. For this reason, its use in rheumatology went slowly and selectively. It took many years before Methotrexate was considered a safe and effective agent that assisted in modifying this disease. This was not easily accomplished; only after years of clinical use was it finally an accepted medication for RA. Even in our new millennium, some Rheumatologists find it difficult to accept it as a frontline treatment.

Methotrexate represents a classic example of how medications grow acceptable. Many times, the manufacturer had been completely unaware that his drug was being used to treat a disease for which it was neither designed, nor approved.

Taking down anecdotal information occasionally may be very useful in medical practice: the early use of Methotrexate is an illustrative example. With no new agents available and the implication that Methotrexate had an effect on a patient's arthritic disease, as well as on his psoriasis, it began being tried sparingly. Not being so-approved, or recognized as an anti-rheumatic agent, it lacked enthusiastic support from many rheumatologists. The agent had been used in the past to a limited extent, but any actual therapeutic dose for arthritis was an unknown. Reports stated it caused cirrhosis of the liver and/or toxic hepatitis. Methotrexate hadn't been used for many years and, as malpractice concerns grew greater and greater, physicians - even its manufacturer - were reluctant to promote its use.

The evolution of Methotrexate as an accepted anti-rheumatic agent was similar to the introduction of Indocin, the first nonsteroidal anti-inflammatory agent. The reason for illustrating this experience is to demonstrate the spiraling around difficulty in selecting new arthritic drugs Rheumatologists faced on their yellow-brick- road towards an RA cure.

Methotrexate was an old drug not a new discovery, but now a new discovery for its use was clear: RA. Soon, it was evident that very active Rheumatoid Arthritis appeared to become quiescent, or even approach remission with Methotrexate. An exciting event was materializing, and clear responses were definitely occurring. Nothing had quieted the disease to this extent since cortisone. Now, greater attention was being paid to assessing how and why this disease could become quiescent and show less activity with Methotrexate. Because of the crude and primitive manner of the drug's introduction, most physicians learned its use individually.

Most arthritis patients, when seen by a Rheumatologist, had received many nonsteroidal agents with even a short course of steroids. The disease usually had progressed enough to be quite active and become a serious management problem. It wasn't unusual for patients to be greatly concerned that they were facing an ominous future of becoming a cripple, and/or needing a joint replaced. The approach to treatment and management of such problems usually progressed to the point that Methotrexate along with additional accompanying agents became the first line of defense. A period of patient and disease management developed where a true positive approach in treatment and control occurred for the first time in dealing with Rheumatoid Arthritis.

The first step in managing acute RA then was to select the joint or joints where the flare-up was most active. One or two of these areas were injected with long-acting corticosteroids, Aristacort (DepoMedrol, cortisone product) mixed with Novocain. If there was a knee or other joint having a large accumulation of joint fluid, aspiration and removal of the synovial fluid was done. This was easily accomplished with one needle insertion. The removal of the aspiration syringe from the needle while the needle remained within the joint space could be easily performed with care. A ten-cc syringe with a number 18-gauge needle was used. After changing syringes with the initial needle still in place, the steroid and Novocain were injected. The patient had been instructed about possible post-injection flare-ups, but with DepoMedrol this was rare. They were counseled that this should offer rather quick, temporary relief of swelling and inflammation. Showing the patient a general diagram of a typical knee joint was instructively helpful in demonstrating where the synovial tissue lay, its proliferation, and potential damaging effect. This procedure of joint aspiration and injection was generally done on the most involved joint and on the occasion of severe inflammation flare-ups. When necessary, two joints could be aspirated and injected during the same visit.

Next the course of Methotrexate utilization and its initial administrated was discussed. The initial mode of choice was intramuscular injection of 7.5 to 10 mgm; the actual amount depended on the patient's size and the disease's severity. In its early use, convincing the patient to take the drug was generally somewhat difficult. As with all the drugs used in Rheumatoid Arthritis treatment, fear accompanies 'what's new', a fear based on earlier experiences, or because of stories about poor results, or adverse effects. It was, nevertheless, very effective and, with the dose and methods used, was found to be relatively safe. Careful close-observation, while this agent was being administered minimized the concern. An original focus on the liver came from prior years reports about cirrhosis being caused by Methotrexate. That complication never materialized with the use of Methotrexate while treating Rheumatoid Arthritis. In fact, it was quite safe. Initial care and diligence surely contributed to the small number of serious side-effects in its early employment. Early on, Methotrexate partially filled the void left by Cortisone.

Any proposed new-plan for treating RA - as was the routine with Methotrexate - is first explained and then closely monitored by a laboratory blood test analysis every two weeks; their testing evaluated basic blood counts, liver, and kidney function. The patient is asked to refrain from all alcohol for the first few months. That restriction was not any concern of an incompatibility in mixing alcohol with Methotrexate, but for minimizing confusing liver-effects. It's known that alcohol can injure the liver and if that were occurring, Methotrexate could be blamed as the cause, and even if Methotrexate is having a positive suppression on the arthritis it would be halted. The patient would then have lost this very effective agent.

There's a valid reason for administration to be by injection: this method removed gastrointestinal absorption as a limiting factor. Injection provides a direct more-effective route to greater bioavailability – meaning, the drug is not altered by GI absorption. Methotrexate is able to have its full effect with the selected dose allowing one to determine if, or how well, it suppressed the activity of the rheumatoid inflammatory process. Dosage effectiveness can best be evaluated as an injectable and later, if desired, oral administration can be substituted. Although injection is the best form of administration, it cannot always be used for a variety of reasons; oral is still a very effective way to use Methotrexate.

It is quite necessary for recipients to understand the concept of bioavailability. When injected, it provides the greatest possible amount of Methotrexate biologically available, and allows it to immediately be infused into the circulation system. When given orally the biological availability [bioavailability] can be limited by gastrointestinal absorption, possibly being further altered by the liver. The goal is to eliminate liver-suspicions by making the Methotrexate as bioavailable as possible in order to determine its inherent effectiveness. Part of its initial program instructed the patient and provided assurance the program is an individually designed treatment.

The first assay in the drug's historical plan was to determine Methotrexate's effect, and the dose needed. Suppressing acute pain in the most involved joints with a steroid injection had once been deemed successful; the program of Methotrexate using this form of injection to suppress or modify RA commenced our customized management of Rheumatoid Arthritis.

While waiting for the Methotrexate to suppress or modify the disease, other assistance in managing RA is generally needed. This is commonly done with any tolerated NSAID's even with an analgesic when needed. The rationalization for such drug intermixtures is that the diminution of synovial proliferation and swelling by steroid-injection; and, beginning with, any earlier-used tolerated anti-inflammatory agents can be very helpful. With this knowledge, one of the NSAID's may be selected to supplement control of the symptoms. The dose is determined by what was used in the past, and the history of tolerance by the GI tract. In order to minimize gastrointestinal problems, an analgesic is also provided, if needed. Darvocet-N or Codeine is often added for pain relief.

This basic program evolved after years of employing Methotrexate to manage Rheumatoid Arthritis. With a variety of doses of and NSAID supported with injectable steroid in symptomatic joints, this could be the first positive feeling that one could truly control this debilitating disease. The fears about devastation that originated with its projected use never came to pass. After years of watching and securing liver function tests, on occasions mildly abnormal liver test results were very rarely found. If detected, they were very rapidly reversed on eliminating Methotrexate. Neither literature nor personal experience has ever reported or witnessed cirrhosis resulting from the amount of Methotrexate used in treating Rheumatoid Arthritis.

As experience progressed, side-effects from this treatment program were minimal to nil. Reasons for elimination included,

- Minimal hair-loss that some women did not want to continue;
- Mild, recurrent viral infections;
- Mild elevation of liver enzymes. (In many years of use, only a few cases were witnessed. Never experienced liver damage. On occasion, this was confused with gall bladder disease, not true drug toxicity);
- Fear of the drug, causing some to refuse it;
- Skin rash, rarely seen;
- Shortness of breath (this appeared to come from fluid retention, or from an allergic reactive response. No long-term problems were seen).

  > It has been recorded that Methotrexate can cause pulmonary fibrosis, but one can dispute this since pulmonary fibrosis is a known problem associated with Rheumatoid Arthritis. This may again be an example of a drug being attached blame for an associated problem but not the true cause.

- Failure to respond.
- Bleeding problems (Rare)

No long-term problems have been encountered with Methotrexate in over a generation. If a problem arose, it was the revelation, over years of use, that it wasn't the panacea it was once considered; it did not cause cirrhosis of the liver as originally cautioned against. Its use elevated management of Rheumatoid Arthritis to another level, offering an agent to control the vast majority of symptoms; this drug was far better than any product from the past, or yet on the scene, for patients with Rheumatoid Arthritis.

Now came an era of positive feeling for treating these diseases. Methotrexate provided a measurable effect in treating and managing Rheumatoid Arthritis. This era followed the excessive caution and fear that preceded the use of this drug. Had it not been for the need to proceed and the courage of patients and physicians, this would not have occurred. In rheumatology at that time, all treatment of RA was literally by trial-and-error. The advanced use of this drug evolved from the trenches where practicing rheumatologist work not from the ivory towers of leaning.

As Methotrexate advanced in usage, it was found to loose effectiveness in long-term use. It ultimately had to be mixed with other DMARD's to further suppress and control Inflammatory Arthritis. The major outgrowth of the added positive treatment of inflamed arthritic joints added further credence to the fact that the traditional programmed treatment-packages were much less meaningful in diagnosing and treating RA than even laboratory studies promulgated. Such tests as rheumatoid factor, antinuclear antibodies, and even x-ray findings were not meaningful in establishing a therapeutic program. This favorable response documented historical findings, coupled to the active physical findings. This demonstrated what the key to diagnoses and treatment was. In Rheumatoid Arthritis, one can punctuate the fact that most clinical information can be gained from four key events:

- How does the patient feel, and what are the present symptoms compared to before the treatment was started?
- How do the involved joints presently appear, and how much active inflammation is present and perceived by a critical physical examination, compared to before the administration of the treatment program?
- How has the treatment worked and, if possible did it improve any abnormality found in the blood work (i.e., sediment rate and/or anemia or white count)?
- Did it improve the patient's quality of life?

This chapter has briefly represented the way Rheumatoid Arthritis is managed and observed with emphasis on the use of Methotrexate, as well as all other modern treatment drugs and procedures that were available then. This era had a unique existence in the history of rheumatology. It began timidly, followed with great expectations, and resulted in noted limitations in effect.

CHAPTER 11
COMMENCING A NEW ERA IN RHEUMATOLOGY

DuPont ads once proclaimed: *"Better living through Chemistry".* In arthritic treatments, we today have: *"Better living through Biochemistry!"*

Rheumatology is entering into its most exciting period yet: to its broad assemblage of disease-modifying agents three, maybe four, new drugs have been added. They appear to be more specific and more effective than any devised in the past. These agents not only offer great promise to Arthritis sufferers, they represent new concepts bringing new insights to management to Rheumatoid Arthritis and other auto-immune diseases.

In considering their long-term effect on Rheumatoid Arthritis, these drugs are in their infancy: much is waiting to be gained by gathering a clear molecular understanding of these drugs, and in learning of dosages appropriate to various patients. Rheumatology has, for years, been treated by applications, physiotherapy, and pain medication, NSAID's and by non-specific immunosuppressive agents. The arthritis field has suddenly entered the molecular immunology arena, and is bringing the immunological medical information into Rheumatology.

Previously little known information on the molecular immunologic activity of inflammation is now being disseminated. This is illustrating and formulating highly specific information on the destructive elements at the joint synovial level. This has resulted in treatment directed at the actual damage mediator, be it infection, trauma, environmental, or genetic. At this writing, the actual causative origin of Inflammatory Arthritis remains unknown although modern molecular biology has identified molecules specifically causing damage to the articular cartilage.

Excitingly to be told, specific agents, for the first time, are being used to alter the synovium against producing such damaging molecular activity. Smith and Haynes[12] have given a unique insight into the new vistas now opening for the treatment of arthritis. In the following précis of such work, please forgive any ultra-technical details; the summary basically demonstrates how biologically deep is the arena of Rheumatology progressing

---

[12] *Smith, J. Bruce and Haynes, Mark K, Rheumatoid Arthritis-A Molecular Understanding, Review, Annals of Internal Medicine, June 2002, Vol.136.No 13*

Smith and Hayes skillfully demonstrate the inflammatory process with the formation of cytokines by proteolytic enzymes, which are induced by pro-inflammatory cytokines, Dayer and Bresnihan[13] also discussed the molecular immunologic activity resulting in extracellular environmental run by proteolytic enzymes; these enzymes are introduced by proinflammatory cytokines, predominately interleukin-1.

This immunological information, which is mentioned, demonstrates the depth of the intellectual immunological knowledge that has developed in Rheumatology. This mountain of molecular immunological data provides correlations to our long-standing clinical appreciation of the destructive nature of synovial inflammation regardless of its underlying cause. Such research is more than just interesting because this corresponds with earlier comments about the origin and cause of osteoarthritis. It has now been demonstrated, more conclusively than ever, that damage originates from molecular substances in the synovium from immunological cells that migrate there, resulting in cartilage damage and ultimately in destruction. This rests well with our theory that most of what is seen as degenerative arthritis is antedated by a mild inflammatory state regardless of its etiology.

In our new era of science and biochemistry, drug manufacturers are designing and manufacturing new biological agents, and directing their activity towards this specific area with precise action - right down to precise molecules. In designing these agents, recommendations are made on side- effects, toxicity, and mode of use. Sadly but realistically to tell, manufacturers do not, and never can, be able to define all there is to know about a drug. True safety and efficacy are only known and determined once a drug has been widely and clinically used.

It ought to be understood that, many manufacturer-claims being purported today are no more exaggerated – and generally far less so - than are the great expectations that precede the releases of non-FDA regulated alternative natural drugs. The newest and most exciting agents will encounter extensive clinical use to determine long-term value and worth.

For an FDA approved drug, expectations occasionally create inappropriate usage problems. As a result, some very effective and valuable preparations have been and are being removed from the market. Even while these new biological agents were coming forth, additional new

---

[13] *Arthritis & Rheumatism, Editorial, Vol 46, No,3 Mar. 2002 pp 574-578, Jean-Michel Dayer and Barry Bresniham, "Targeting Interleukin-1 in the treatment of Rheumatoid Arthritis."*

and innovative NSAID's had arrived. However, past mistakes were unfortunately disregarded.

A classic and previously noted example of one such mistake was Lilly's anti-inflammatory Oraflex. This had been released with a great deal of media-hype and dreamy-expectation. Oraflex even claimed to effect some reversal of Rheumatoid Arthritis bone erosions. Patients, on hearing about such manufacturer's claims and wanting to try Oraflex, were daily calling Rheumatologists. Its market-stay lasted almost a month. If the same circumstances had prevailed when we were working with Indocin twenty-five years earlier, Indocin would never have come on the market. We now have some exceptionally good agents to control the severe inflammatory process. There would be more if one could interest manufactures into concentrating on improving what is already available now, while implementing better methods to administer and monitor treatment.

Our present Rheumatological era might come to be viewed as an epoch while agents that are more meaningful are becoming available along with ever-greater understanding of the disease's mechanics amid continued research on the structure and active mechanism of these agents. Excitement best describes today's Rheumatology.

There presently are four very momentous agents for treating and controlling Rheumatoid Arthritis - with a fifth remaining questionable. Some study into altering and modifying the ease with which they are administered would be of benefit to each of them. In the past, the manufacturer developed dose and administration procedures, and presented them to the clinician. In the future, subsequent clinical monitoring of actual chemical effect and dosage adjustment with respect to individual patients will help in using many newer drugs.[3]This aspect of drug dosing and utilization arise from clinical management not from the manufacturer regardless the trials antedating release of them.

The new biological drugs are worthwhile, effective, and well researched. All this being present, we shall now attempt to introduce them, illustrate their use, and describe their effectiveness. Safety having become the dominant concern, treating and managing Arthritis has been fully changed. The first drug to be mentioned may justifiably exemplify this: it has had some destructive biological effects. Nevertheless, this no-longer-available agent does indicate promise in treating non-pregnant women; we use it to illustrate a biological area of action similar to the new agents used in treatment.

THALIDOMIDE

"Thalidomide[14.15.] was synthesized in Germany in 1954 as part of a program to develop new antihistamines for the treatment of allergy. Subsequent testing showed this new compound to be a relatively poor antihistamine, but it did turn out to be an effective hypnotic (Note 1), a drug capable of inducing drowsiness and sleep.

However, it now appears that the principal mechanism of thalidomide's anti-inflammatory effectiveness is its ability to inhibit the production of the cytokine tumor necrosis factor alpha (TNF-α), a potent stimulator of inflammation. Normally found in barely detectable amounts, the levels of TNF-α rise dramatically in chronic inflammatory conditions. The cytokine thus appears to sustain inflammation beyond the point at which it can become harmful; indeed, TNF-α is now known to be a principal mediator of the deadly toxic shock that develops in response to some bacterial infection.

"Thalidomide effectively shuts down the production of TNF-α by inhibiting its production in monocytes and macrophages. Represented here is another modern example at the direction toward the TNF-α in the inflammatory process and drugs related."

Thalidomide is in disrepute but has the potential to treat the molecular immunological state of Rheumatoid Arthritis. Using newer agents that have greater specificity does not preclude traveling the same route tried years ago, specifically disease-modifying agents in using combinations with various doses. While acquiring greater knowledge of these and even older drugs, we may be cutting new pathways. Is it not surprising how an agent such as Kineret, which should have blocked inflammation, was

---

[14.] A Background Briefing by Dennis Blakeslee, PhD .is a start .at discussing this agent. (Posted January 29, 1998) This site produced by the Journal of the American Medical Association.

[15.] *Thalidomide is the same drug removed from the market because of birth deformities.*

clinically ineffective, while Thalidomide[15] an antihistamine, may prove effective as an anti-inflammatory? Examples like these demonstrate the necessity for close clinical cooperation between the treating physician and the pharmaceuticals manufacturer.

Because of Thalidomide's effect on TNF-α which is presently recognized as the molecular substance and culprit considered damaging to cartilage; this drug may find a future in treating inflammatory diseases. Our present drugs do have all the appearance of being a panacea; however there has not been a sufficient clinical use to assure this. Hopefully, if time overcomes the dastardly congenital defects this drug caused by its inappropriate use as a sleeping pill in pregnant women, it may have a helpful future; it is an inexpensive oral agent targeting the same substances as the nearly cost-prohibitively new biological drugs. It should find a specific place in management of inflammatory joint disease. The major problem remains that clinical trials in today's society almost make this impossible; physicians and manufacturers will loath encountering liability risk in today's environment. Without attempting to study a specific drug in patients with a disease, it seems its efficacy will never be known. Very limited experience with this agent illustrates it is effective in autoimmune diseases.

New advances in treating Rheumatoid Arthritis are attacking its rudiment: its physiological mechanics. An entirely novel concept has been introduced: developing anti-Tumor-Necrosis-Factor-alpha technology.

The triggering event or agent initiating or causing Rheumatoid Arthritis remains unknown, but for years, we had been without any new chemical or any potential modifying advance for treating this disease. The advent of new agents – even if they carried unreadable complex chemical names – came a new approach to advancing against the disease. Interleukins having been discussed for years, our thought processes were stimulated into thinking about how our treatments evolved. Most of this immunology was hypothetical research so it was believed that any actual management at this biochemical level would not occur in our lifetime. So for years, all new agents were not new concepts just another creation. Then came Arava, Kineret, Enbrel, and Remicade and more.

ARAVA

This new oral agent[v] arrived sans flourish. It was established to alter the immune system's hyperactivity: aiming to manage and treat Rheumatoid

---

[v] The second drug to be effective but not flourish in the new treatment era

Arthritis specifically. This succeeding Technical Description is for illustrative purposes to show how much our profession is medically progressing from this new agent aggregate.

In biologic terms, Arava, or leflunomide, is an isoxazole immunomodulatory agent that inhibits dihydroorotate dehydrogenase (an enzyme involved in de-novo pyrimidine synthesis), and has antiproliferative activity. Several in-vivo and in-vitro experimental models have demonstrated an anti-inflammatory effect. These chemical descriptions intricately illustrate the depth of research that has gone into seeking answers in the advance on Rheumatoid Arthritis. We have taken the progress on the inflammatory pharmacokinetics to a deeper, more primitive level by reaching into the recesses of its causative phenomenon. The pharmaceutical action of Arava is stated as:

> *"Following oral administration, leflunomide is metabolized to an active metabolite A77 1726 (hereafter referred to as M1), which is responsible for essentially all of its activity in vivo. Plasma levels of leflunomide are occasionally seen, at very low levels. Studies of the pharmacokinetics of leflunomide have primarily examined the plasma concentrations of this active metabolite."*

Arava was released in 1998 as a new agent to control the disease better: one superior to Methotrexate. Up to then in the previous twenty years, Methotrexate had been our major control drug. Arava appears to offer another phase for controlling rheumatic diseases.

It is an oral agent agreeably administered - pharmaceutical companies generally direct how their drugs should be administered. In the period of Gold, Plaquenil, and Methotrexate, the manufacturer knew nothing about drugs being used in managing rheumatoid and inflammatory diseases. Then it was clinical experience that determined how, and how much of these earlier drugs were used.

A major problem of management with Arava was manifested on its arrival. The original dosing samples called for loading the system with 100 mgm a day for three days, because biochemical analysis determined that Arava was protein-bound, not bioavailable until it was fully bound to plasma protein. Following this, a maintenance dose of 20 mgm was recommended. This test-tube-concept appeared reasonable, however this was not a practical method of utilization for an active rheumatic patient: whose fine end-point detects the effect of an anti-rheumatic agent.

The drug at the outset was a quite satisfactory agent to treat Rheumatoid Arthritis. Early in its use its most limiting factor was diarrhea.

In some instances, it can be quite disabling so, when it occurs, the drug was discontinued. The problem of diarrhea turned out to be the major limiting factor in its use. This was not brought up in alerts from the manufacturer. It ought to have been stressed as an occurrence and investigated for possible ways of controlling and not become a major reason for cessation of use. In searching out the causative mechanism of the diarrhea, even the manufacturer[16.] could not provide an answer as to why it occurs with Arava. Since Arava is a very promising for arthritis, the cause should and be determined – unless it is withdrawn from fear of litigation. That would be arthritis' great loss. Knowing as much as possible about the systemic cause behind the diarrhea might assist in its administration and handling of the compound. As shown before, diarrhea is not exclusive to Arava; many good drugs own this side effect.

Many such patients were immediately excluded from using the recommended dose because the high loading doses provoked early undesirable side effects before the desired therapeutic effect was able to manifest itself. In addition smaller doses might well have been effective and/or useful with other agents to treat Inflammatory Arthritis.

BEFORE DISCUSSING OUR FOUR NEWEST BIOLOGICAL DRUGS, ONE MUST INTRODUCE IMPORTANT SIDE ISSUES?

In the past, individual dosing of arthritic medicines was very much a trial-and-error situation. These patients have a great personal, not literature-ability in determining whether that drug was having its claimed effect. If pain, swelling, and stiffness are better, these drugs are going to be used. Therefore, if it is to be effective in assessing a treatment for RA, the selected dose is easily determined. These days, this is not a common phenomenon with new drugs and agents in medicine.

Because of our litigious society, both physicians and drug houses are oversensitive to drug doses and to side effects. Almost all patients will have diarrhea with the recommended loading dose of Arava. The protocol offers little, and no, variability with dosing. As a result, neither the manufacturer nor the physicians using the drug are able to evaluate the full effect of the drug, or its true status, or its potency for suppressing Rheumatoid Arthritis. All drugs are effective at variable dose levels for different persons because of the individuality of Rheumatoid Arthritis. The standard manufacturers' recommended doses are sometimes neither totally realistic nor always effective. Individuality of the disease causes arthritic

---

[16.] *Avitis, the manufacturer, was called April 10, 2002 in order to find and answer to the diarrhea. They could not provide the answer.*

responses to a standard dose unsuitable. It is not unusual for the most effective doses to be half or double the original recommended dose. Occasionally, when combined with other agents, there can be an added effect to alter a dosage. This was common in the past when a wide variety of drugs were used and mixed. Varied methods of drug utilization and patient management were stopped when drug houses suggested every one of the potential problems and potential side effects. Also, many times over the years varied doses and in combination with other disease modifying agents are found tolerable and effective. This never happened while Arava was being used more extensively.

Dealing with immunological diseases having no known cause, and a wide clinical variety - including Rheumatoid Arthritis - can be very confusing, especially with so many new biological management procedures.

Consider the broad prospect of potential viral infestations and virus-like infections in light of all the marketing documentation being disseminated to us. This is well illustrated in Madeline Drexel's book, "Secret Agents, The Menace of Emerging Infections". Her manuscript describes the difficulty by picturing documentation of disseminated viral diseases unless there is suspicion and investigation. The diseases discussed are those that present nonspecific lethal results, fever, liver and kidney failure, and bone marrow suppression.

Hypersensitive reactions or drug idiosyncrasies have similar presentations: some had been described early in this manuscript. It is possible that such diseases and infections can be blamed on the drugs being used. False trials can creates problems that are onerous in a clinical situation where occasionally a more natural effect is attributed to a good and effective drug. The same difficulty arises in assigning clinically effective doses to these and other drugs. Critical clinical acumen remains important in managing rheumatic diseases using both old and new drugs.

De-facto use of new anti-rheumatic drugs – or any new drug - requires years of clinical observation before its definitively therapeutic efficacy, safety, and actions are understood with precision. Early pronouncements from a manufacturer are almost never factual. Promoting and marketing is counterproductive: for this reason and others *'public advertising of drugs should be prohibited'!*

As previously mentioned, all therapeutic agents have wide and varied results: some are not all good; none are all bad [consider thalidomide or nicotine]. People being protein individuals, responses to drugs are just as individual as are multifaceted DNA persons. What is needed in using and assessing drugs is a long-term, careful clinical observation while carefully monitoring therapeutic regimens, as well as continual education about the disease being treated.

Rheumatology has a number of powerful new anti-rheumatic drugs, but practicing Rheumatologists are not provided with enough time to knowledgeably formulate good clinical-judgments concerning them. The latest potent drugs for Rheumatoid Arthritis have only been used for only over four years. It is far too early to know all their clinical activity and effects.

There are other new agents - completely unknown to the majority of physicians - being used to treat Rheumatoid Arthritis. These and their future generations are potentially the-most-powerful agents for treating hypersensitivity (autoimmune) diseases for which we still cannot establish a definitive cause: Arthritis is only one of near thirty named such autoimmune diseases. These drugs and the ones they precede need a great deal of clinical experience and time to determine if they provide the best result.

Treating Inflammatory Arthritis frequently necessitates experimenting with multiple drugs and combinations in a wide variety of individual doses. The treatment of this form of arthritis actually is done via trial-and-error. Any new drug must be made available to enough patients in a clinically reliable study. Combining an interested, compassionate physician with informed patients-in-need provides anchors to truly assess the ability of a new agent to alter the course of Rheumatoid Arthritis.

As previously noted, individuals of the legal community are already advertising about problems with Arava. Who dare assume that all is clinically and chemically known in every patient with Rheumatoid Arthritis who have used Arava during the relatively short time it's been around.

Arava was the most effective anti-rheumatic drug in the last three decades. In a fashion most remarkable, this oral drug [and its associated-drugs] dramatically decreased inflammation in severely active Rheumatoid Arthritis. No treatment since Methotrexate had the therapeutic effect Arava produced. Obviously, many patients did not respond favorably; the reasons 'why not' need further clinical observation and consideration. Experience with other drugs reveals a variety of assessments are needed. With other therapies, a variety of doses and combinations were utilized; Arava was not given such a chance. Time for such effort was not permitted, nor was it given the liberty other drugs had in treating Rheumatoid Arthritis.

KINERET

Kineret was released as the first drug to address the disease, Rheumatoid Arthritis at its origin to attack a damage-causative agency. It was intended to block a specific molecular agent that was causing the inflammation of Rheumatoid Arthritis. (Data from the manufacturer)

Kineret™[17.] Thousand Oaks, Caliph, Amgen Inc.; 2001

"The pathogenesis of Rheumatoid Arthritis is a complex process that leads to significant and chronic joint inflammation. Interleukin-1 (IL-1) is a central mediator in Rheumatoid Arthritis and is a critical proinflammatory cytokine that has been found to be abundant in the synovial fluid of RA patients.

"IL-1 and TNF-_ are thought to share several biologic actions. IL-1 and TNF-α induce the production of each other, and they act synergistically. Experimental human peripheral blood and animal model systems have shown TNF-α induces IL-1, IL-1 induces TNF-α. These are the specific molecular agents that are involved in and being credited as substances that cause damage in RA.

"Interleukin's role in the events in Rheumatoid Arthritis (RA) and the IL–1 are stated by the manufacturer of Kineret: the key concepts are as follows:

IL-1 has been shown to be a dominant cytokine associated with RA.

IL-1 production is induced in response inflammatory stimuli and mediates various physiologic responses including inflammatory and immunological responses.

IL-1 has a broad range of activities including cartilage degradation by its induction of the rapid loss of proteoglycans, as well as stimulation of bone resorption."

This bio-chemical molecular-immunological investigation resulted in manufacturing a drug that specifically attacked this immune system. It was

---

[17.] *Kineret™ [prescribing information]. Thousand Oaks, Calif, Amgen Inc.; 2001.*

made by Amgen and marketed as 'Kineret'. In all respects, it should have been a very effective drug in treating and managing Rheumatoid Arthritis. Clinically, not all of this promise materialized metabolically. Kineret did not arrest or have a legitimate clinical effect on active Rheumatoid Arthritis. All of this huge biological investigation coupled with the large expenditure of manufacturing and marketing this drug to block interleukin-1, which it did, unfortunately was like picking the wrong horse in the race (IL-1).

The well-illustrated chemical biological molecular immunology of the workings of Kineret was very logical but it was clinically ineffective. Unless further assessment of this agent is made, what appears to be an interesting drug may fall totally out of use. In all probability, it could be an agent that needs to be associated with other inflammation treatments. Kineret illustrates how test-tube-logic does not always materialize when used clinically. On the other hand, some very old drugs not so test-tube considered do unexpectedly succeed with arthritics.

A new use for old drugs is not uncommon in medicine. Many of today's very effective drugs were originally developed for other, often entirely unrelated purposes, decades after its introduction as an analgesic, aspirin was found to be a highly potent antithrombotic agent. Prozac and its relatives, serotonin reuptake inhibitors, were first marketed as appetite suppressants. Minoxidil, an antihypertensive agent, is now marketed to treat baldness. The fungal antibiotics, cyclosporine and lovostatin, were later found to have additional effects, cyclosporine as the key to transplantation; lovostatin as a cholesterol-lowering agent.

ENBREL

Immunex Corporation [Seattle, WA] developed the anti-tumor necrosis factor, Enbrel (Etanercept). It was genetically engineered as a biological response modifier and represents a novel approach to the management of patients with active Rheumatoid Arthritis. Enbrel was then the most specific drug being directed at the TNF-α using anti-TNF-α to treat rheumatoid Inflammatory Arthritis. This special agent is of human-antibody origin. It is fabricated by fusing two naturally occurring soluble TNF-receptors making it resemble a protein that the body produces naturally. The production of this agent is expensive and time consuming.

Recognizing TNF-α as the central player in the pathophysiology in Rheumatoid Arthritis led to developing a new class of agents, anti-TNF-α drugs. For the first time in generations, pharmaceutical companies began developing drugs for Rheumatoid Arthritis. Manufacturers were concerned about these disease-modifying agents' indiscriminately suppressing the immune system. That could cause trouble in patients handling exposure to infection, placing them at risk. This utmost concern was a major limiting factor in anti-TNF-α drugs.

When considering the use of Enbrel and similar drugs, Rheumatologists now specify an agent with a specific biochemical-known effect. With this greater responsibility having been added to management, our discipline began moving – out of necessity - away from its primitive era of rheumatology - injecting strep vaccines blindly affecting the immune system – elevating to true modern treatment specificity. In the past, trial-and-error treatment – often with total unknown effect - prevailed as an active mode: the heavy use of Gold injection being one example. The scene now advanced to injecting anti-Tumor Necrosis Factor-alpha. Before utilizing a treatment, Rheumatologists needed to think and consider what the drug company had produced and how it purported to work. It was reported that Enbrel (anti-TNF-α) binds TNF-α as well as lymphotoxin-α. This obviously created a legitimate concern about the patient's defense mechanism against infection.

As this treatment was enthusiastically considered a very positive new treatment approach for Inflammatory Arthritis, another barrier was encountered. This extremely promising drug had all the biochemical structure and activity to legitimately treat this disease, but cost was a factor. In treating a disease, where patients will try almost anything to quiet pain, Enbrel was eagerly anticipated. Concern for side effects may have been excessive because of present day attitudes; however, cost was its most limiting factor. The public was reluctantly accepting expensive drugs at $3.00 to $4.00 a pill, but the expensive monthly cost of Enbrel that was being projected at $1,300 was unacceptable for most. In addition, it is always legitimate to ask how long the treatment was to continue, and the logical explanation was, until the disease improved and that was unknown. Knowing the history of Rheumatoid Arthritis, this meant an indefinite period. High-cost was a major problem negating the drug's institution. Most insurance companies would not reimburse that drug-cost. All of these factors: unknown potential side effects; unknown duration of treatment; self injection; and high cost made, at the outset, Enbrel's administration very difficult.

In covering the entire spectrum, clinical observation was, at first, quite mixed. At its initial introduction - as with all new agents – came an expectation that a definitive cure may finally have arrived.

Since it is initially dedicated to the most active and aggressive cases, the response is usually most gratifying. Soon, additional responses are less dramatic, and it was found that using Methotrexate with

There is no reliable rationale for such reasoning. If the drug is effective, but will not sustain its therapeutic effect, there is less chance for the effect to be enhanced for a longer time with a larger dose. First, the larger dose exposes its patient to more of the chemical compound, which increases the risk for accumulation and/or toxic effect. By shortening the interval, one takes advantage of a known clinical response: an ability to keep the disease under control as it is being suppressed by a lower dose. This concept is unacceptable to the insurance carriers.

The manufacturer did not originally support this clinical observation either, which implies that the suggested dose is frequently inadequate. Efforts to have the manufacturer substantiate the need for shorter intervals were in the beginning to no avail. In the past, drugs were produced and the clinician had the responsibility, and the latitude, to determine - and report - the value and strength of the agent. The process was not limited by fear of litigation. It generally takes considerable time to truly evaluate the effectiveness and potency of any specific drug. It is not uncommon to have a drug intended for one treatment program to find use in another. Examples previously noted are Plaquenil for malaria and Methotrexate for leukemia. It does appear, however, that the manufacturer of Remicade has modified its insistence on its originally recommended dosing.

HUMIRA

Shortly after the above drug releases, Abbott Laboratories developed the third anti-TNF-α drug to treat Rheumatoid Arthritis. This unique biological drug evolved into a new treatment category. Now we had three biologically different agents, each having its own unique administering routine. Each, however, was directed at the same molecular binding of TNF-α; and each was manufactured differently. This now broadened the choice of drug and illustrated the variety of effect from these agents.

Humira (adalimumab) is also a human-biologically manufactured monoclonal antibody. The manufacturer promotes it as the first human monoclonal antibody approved for reducing signs and symptoms by inhibiting the progression of structural joint and cartilage damage (in adults with moderately to severely active Rheumatoid Arthritis).

This statement by Abbott suggests we may have more such drugs in the future. Biological therapy - referred to as immunotherapy or biotherapy - employs biologic response modifiers (BRM's). These are supposed to stimulate or restore the immune system's ability to fight disease. These make up entirely new considerations in terminology as well as now understanding a cause of the inflammatory process. Gone went our simplistic approaches of just relieving pain, and trying to diminish joint inflammation with an injection; then waiting for relief, or even blocking the damaging agents with much less specific drugs.

Humira is also different in that it is 40 mgm administered subcutaneously every two weeks, making it very competitive with the other anti-TNF-α agents. Since these three biological drugs: Enbrel, Remicade, and Humira are structurally different, it seems clinically obvious that some patients will respond differently. Happily, this does broaden the therapeutic prospective for a Rheumatoid Arthritis patient.

The biochemical action, again is a very technical description, of this newest anti-TNF-α has its own unique activity mode as described by the manufacturer, Abbott:

> *"Adalimumab (Humira) binds specifically to TNF-α and blocks its interaction with the p55 and p75 cell surface TNF-α receptors. Adalimumab also lyses surface TNF-α expressing cells in vitro in the presence of complement. Adalimumab does not bind or inactivate lymphotoxin (TNF-β). TNF-α is a naturally occurring cytokine that is involved in normal inflammatory and immune responses."*

> *It is worthy of restating the purpose of these drugs is that they are acting on elevated levels of the molecule TNF-α found in the synovial membrane and fluid of RA patients. These biological drugs play an important role in treating both pathologic inflammation and joint cartilage destruction: the hallmarks of Rheumatoid Arthritis. This drug Humira now represents another anti-TNF-α drug for the treatment of Rheumatoid Arthritis. Abbott the manufacture further states:*

> *"After treatment with anti-TNF-α, a rapid decrease in levels of acute phase reactants of inflammation (C-reactive protein (CRP) and erythrocyte sedimentation rate (ESR) and serum cytokines (IL-6) was observed compared to baseline in patients with Rheumatoid Arthritis. Serum levels of matrix metalloproteinases (MMP-1 and MMP-3) that produce tissue remodeling responsible for cartilage destruction were also decreased after anti-TNF-α, administration."*

All of this means is if the day arrives that some of these immunologic substances could be measured clinically and the correct dose of anti-TNF-α could be administered to block TNF-α the Inflammatory Arthritis treatment could be titrated according to the need of each individual patient.

There are now, three recognized clinically effective anti-TNF-α agents which have made treatment of Rheumatoid Arthritis eminently successful and, for the first time in the last half-century, aimed at a very specific target.

It is early, but there is a great deal to learn about these drugs. Already the first adverse effect - limiting utilization - is a cumulative allergic reaction developing in some. This creates a critical management problem. With the general very positive effective treatment using these agents, allergies necessitates altering the drug or accepting it potential stoppage either in the patient or in a court. This is correlated to the magnitude of the allergy and its persistence of increased degree. We are experiencing a new birth in treating inflammation and arthritis. There is much to be learned. Still, it appears to be certain that Rheumatology patients' future is as promising as Rheumatology's future is exciting.

*G*reat was the promise occurring on developing anti-TNF-α therapy [with Enbrel, Humira & Remicade], the vista for Rheumatology was far-reaching. This new and innovative modern-time treatment was the greatest advance in controlling and quieting this disease; it is, however, saddled with unheralded limitations. Past therapeutic agents and drugs had been introduced with suggested doses not mandated dosings since it was understood and accepted that it takes time to ascertain strengths and potencies for technological groundbreaking compounds. Along with cutting this uncharted path, no note was given of the hard-learned understanding that all persons act and respond differently to drugs as uniquely as they do to their diseases. Patient and disease have to be individually managed with a special amount of the specific agent selected for the individual's treatment. It was patient management with measured treatment, not disease management, which is today's treatment dictum.

Here is our present case: at all levels, treatment has changed! Nothing illustrates this better than an arthritis' novel "anti-TNF-α Therapy" for Rheumatoid Arthritis. With all the new and rapid diagnostic tools available today: CT scans, MRIs, specific chemical tests, and visualization of organs using scopes and angiograms to formulate specific diagnoses, the history of the patient's symptoms and physical findings seem to be considered irrelevant. This is not the case.

At the same time, immunologic diseases are having specific therapeutic agents developed for their various tissues that are damaged. Some early examples of this were precisely in this field of rheumatology. For example: on being discovered, Penicillin was found to kill bacteria such as streptococcus bacteria thereby eliminating rheumatic fever caused by strep toxins. Allopurinol was discovered to block the purine metabolism of uric acid, thereby fully controlling gout.

Now, with several new biological drugs as like Enbrel, Remicade, and Humira in hand, there is molecular anti-TNF-α therapy in the treatment of Rheumatoid Arthritis. With these drugs the indications in treating RA (Inflammatory Arthritis) are so unambiguous, and the treatment so specific that the treatment program seems almost like a cookbook application. The agents are manufactured for these special diseases and prescribed with the recommended treatment doses has changed treatment patterns.

Cookbookery actions now seem in control of medicine, such examples are:

- Medical students are taught to treat diseases;
- Drug houses create precise biochemical compounds for these diseases propounding and promoting specific doses for the each disease. (Remicade has an explicit dose for Rheumatoid Arthritis and another one for Crohn's disease.) ;
- Insurance companies and HMOs cover the cost of treating diseases, and prior approval for many is now mandated;
- Diagnostic codes used for diseases almost always sound ambiguous while being related to the specific patient.

Our present scheme of so-called "Health Care", leaves the patient entirely out of the equation and the physician, being nowhere mentioned or considered, is abdicated from control. Patient consideration is patently dismissible. Lost is the understanding that illness and disease act differently in dissimilar people. Their presentation can be different, and with the course of their disease behaving unlike all others. In learning about and practicing therapy, came the realization that in the course of treating a disease the required dose of medication differs from patient to patient, with a wide range of variables being involved. Modern medicine however tends to treat diseases under a concept of 'Disease Management'. This poses the dilemma facing modern treatment, especially anti-TNF-α therapy, which - as stated earlier – mandates customized individual patient management.

In their actions against the use of this anti-TNF-α therapy, HMOs and insurance companies have a reasonably understood critique: it's too expensive! [And the next generation of immunologic biochemicals will likely be more so.] To countermand this legitimate claim, manufacturer and physicians must undertake to defend the demonstrable successful treatments with these drugs, and responsibly educate the agency paying for the drug that present payment with a payback from lower future costs. The therapeutic concern is a need for variability of dosage. It has been almost impossible to invoke the manufacturers to accept the need for allowing variability in utilizing anti-TNF-α therapy. As had been mentioned, lost is the treatment of patients, by focusing merely upon a generality: disease management.

Remicade's manufacturer, Centocor, was originally most difficult in failing to accept that physician-indicating dose and interval actually varies from patient to patient but, today after taking a great deal of time in acquiescing to the obvious, Centocor fully understands that variability by publicly stating that the dose and administration interval of Remicade can vary dramatically from patient to patient – even if it's yet to be stated in their distribution protocol.

The same forfeiture of responsibility rests with Immunex, the manufacturer of Enbrel. These companies have created an area of treatment that's near impossible to alter. In treating these potent and quite specific hypersensitivity diseases does require an entirely new approach. Unfortunately in inventing this modality, they are abdicating one of a number of very critical areas. Pharmaceutical houses should be supporting physicians using their new technologies, especially anti-TNF-α therapy because of its specificity and uniqueness. Its agents carry aspects that even their manufacturers are unaware of, such as the effect it has on hypersensitivity diseases, and patient tolerability. Even now, there's much to be learned here. The autoimmunity name alone means self and immunity indicating that an antibody's activity is individual not universal. What could be more illuminating?

Those with courage and knowledge of treating Rheumatoid Arthritis and autoimmune diseases must acknowledge that doses recommended by manufacturers' need not be made sacrosanct since they cannot fit all patients. Already, many are collectively utilizing the drugs individually to discover their full impact in treating severe cases of Rheumatoid Arthritis. Arava is, and has been, used to manage some patients. Enbrel and Arava combinations have been used; altered doses of each have been considered and used. Even minor DMARD combinations have been added in desperate attempts to manage some patients. Since the release of the anti-TNF-α, Methotrexate has been suggested as a complement in treatment.

One of the most bothersome areas for treatments is the dosing of Remicade. Almost no one can be well maintained on the manufacturer's recommended dosage. Most of the rationale behind its unwillingness to defend its attitude concerning doses is corporate not patient protection. Protecting themselves against lawsuits rather than being concerned about the place these agents have in future care of Rheumatoid Arthritis patient-care dominates their thinking.

Here are two examples of what might be called unconventional treatment of Rheumatoid Arthritis with an indiscriminate use of new drugs, and anti TNF-α therapy:

1. An elderly Rheumatoid Arthritis patient on such a treatment regimen that required Methotrexate, Arava, and Enbrel, with three mgm of prednisone for disease control. This patient, when originally seen, had numerous stomach bleeding episodes from gastritis and ulcers. Aspirin and all the known NSAID's were subsequently tried more than once, resulting in major intolerance and ultimately, bleeding.

Out of desperation, doubled acceptable doses of gold and of Methotrexate were utilized; even large doses of Arava were ineffective. After much trial-and-error, the most acceptable program was Methotrexate, Arava, and Enbrel. This was a very drastic use of combined agents. With this most untraditional - and probably non-recommended – program, it was the first time in more than 20 years of unrelenting, aggressive, damaging Rheumatoid Arthritis that this patient felt like a happy, comfortable person. In time steroids and Arava were eliminated and the Methotrexate dose was diminished.

2. A Rheumatoid Arthritis patient, living with a very aggressive disease that was manifested by severe multiple joint swelling, pain and inflammation, was in the early stages of severe damage. After trying all the drugs and traditional modalities available, the patient gave up all, and the disease flared. The programs being administered were gold, Methotrexate, Arava and a variety of combinations supplemented with oral and intra-articular steroids. The RA had originally responded to Arava, however near intolerable diarrhea associated with a severe rash were its side effects. Arava could not be tolerated in combinations with other DMARD's or small doses of Arava.

Enbrel originally also produced a very good response but that resulted in unspecified upper respiratory allergic reactions and, after a few weeks, it began losing effectiveness. Remicade's protocol designs it to be administered every eight weeks. Initially instituted treatment in this patient was extremely effective, but after six weeks of a near full suppression of inflammation, a severe flare resulted. A full reactivation of the Rheumatoid Arthritis occurred, requiring large steroid doses to control and suppress that activity. Attempts to establish a program of Methotrexate in a fairly full dose was tried since the patient's HMO did not allow a six-week normal amount of Remicade.

Desperately, after six weeks on Remicade which had lost its effect, the patient on her own administered 25 mgm of Enbrel subcutaneously every five days or so for the last two weeks. After an estimated few months of her program of alternating Remicade for six weeks and Enbrel during the other two, the patient had the best anti-rheumatic control ever achieved in ten or twelve years of her active, aggressive Rheumatoid Arthritis. In time, her disease was controlled with a slightly larger dose of Remicade supplemented with small doses of Enbrel as needed.

These are anecdotal examples of desperate patients who dare try anything to suppress their diseases. Patient and physician need an understanding of the uniqueness of these hypersensitivity diseases, and a willingness to individualize treatments with the consent and understanding of the patient serious risks may exist. Such anecdotal examples are quite representative of Rheumatoid Arthritis patients.

Having annotated modern pharmacy's dosage problems, we may now bring forth another problem area of modern pharmaceutical activity, one that's neither good for the patient nor for our industry itself: **Public Advertising!** New drug ads, especially those of anti-TNF-α agents are not only not helpful, they are counterproductive. The manufacturers of the drugs Enbrel, Humira, and Remicade, are spending millions to advertise on television, in magazines, and in newspapers. In the past, most advertising was in medical journals, medical meetings, and doctor's offices – now the latter is approaching non-existence.

The manufacturers of these effective new-drugs, Immunex, Centocor, Abbott, and Avitis exhaust millions of dollars on ads directed toward people with arthritis. These promotions are doctrinaire in many aspects concerning their offerings, and anti-TNF-α therapy. Many physicians and all potential patients have little or no knowledge about the drugs, though Rheumatologists have considerable knowledge for utilizing this therapy. The three manufacturers of these drugs are directing their publicity towards patients having a demonstrated predilection for chasing after miracle cures ranging from herbs to acupuncture. This provokes two cost-effectiveness questions, the propriety of spending so lavishly; and where is the message going?

While companies are deluging the airwaves, the number of rheumatologists is diminishing. There is no outcry against such advertising but there are those in the medical profession who take umbrage with respect to this activity.

The path we are traveling along will produce newer, more powerful and more scientifically specific drugs, needing as much in skilled physicians and specialties. Instead of these pharmaceuticals hurling all this money on TV spots, on magazine ads and at lobbyists, they ought to be directing funds towards rheumatologists' fellowship training. Medical schools need Professors interested in this specialty. Their rheumatology department head has usually been a research physician or immunologist who's not really interested in clinical arthritis, or in treating arthritis patients.

A third problem facing our industry is the tendency to sue large companies when a complaint is made. This tends to make pharmaceutical companies sensitive about how they release, or if they release, or to whom they release their drugs. It was never that way in the past. Let's study Methotrexate as an example of a good drug early on being charged falsely. Sometimes it seems that to suppress a disease is less important that in suppressing an agent, which suppresses the disease:

Methotrexate is now the first line of defense as a disease-modifying agent. It is very effective in suppressing and controlling Inflammatory Arthritis. Its use had been devised via a trial-and- error method long before it was released and approved for RA by the FDA. The actual dose administered to control RA was patient-determined as had occurred in most drugs in treating arthritis. A general maintenance dose varies between 7.5 and 15 mgm a week, although some use higher doses. Prior to Methotrexate use in severe cases, there was great fear of the toxicity to the liver but cirrhosis of the liver has not proven itself a known side-effect in the treatment of Rheumatoid Arthritis.

Methotrexate has also been wrongly incorrectly incriminated for causing pulmonary fibrosis from a suggestion of its enhancement of pulmonary fibrosis due to Methotrexate, but that was a mere conjecture. It is historically well known that exaggerated pulmonary response is due to exogenous stimuli. The most well known historical documentation is the Caplan's Syndrome. This was the first true observation of pulmonary disease and its connection with Rheumatoid Arthritis. It was first reported in Welsh coal miners. Caplan, in screening x-rays of miners discovered large pulmonary nodules. He further discovered that these miners had Rheumatoid Arthritis. He concluded that the lungs of miners with rheumatoid disease were hypersensitive to the stimulus of coal dust, which was causing their pulmonary nodules.

Methotrexate should not be cavalierly implicated as a potential agent enhancing the proclivity for fibrosis of a rheumatoid lung. A high index of suspicion ought be assigned to allegations carrying no factual evidence linking some effect to a presumed cause [that's how science works, but that's why a courtroom uses words not data?]. Nevertheless, while using Methotrexate, one must constantly be cognizant of respiratory complaints. In reference to respiratory problems, cause-and-effect does not a correlate definitively. After a generation of using Methotrexate, it has proven very effective, and a safe agent for suppressing Rheumatoid Arthritis.

With cul-de-sac obstacles help to patient relief having been set out a route to expunction, let's return to helpful patient care:

Rheumatoid (inflammatory) Arthritis treatment has climbed to a uniquely different level. This inflammatory disease is being acquitted of its old prognosis as an incurable and totally crippling disease with no effective treatments. It's now a disease with a wide variety of treatment options, with the options expanding in number, nature, and technology! In the past, one picked one or two drugs and planned on slowly adding additional forms of treatment, as each response inevitably grew inadequate. Rheumatology's present mindset is to suppress it aggressively, after evaluating the inflammatory state and its severity. The best approach is to determine whether one can obliterate the process with drugs that are suitable and tolerable, rather than prod at the problem.

To accomplish this, one must proceed in an orderly fashion in managing the inflammatory joint disease. The first temporary step is to overwhelm the inflammation in the affected joint(s) with a local injection in the most violently involved areas using a long-acting steroid. Next, is to begin with an oral anti-inflammatory agent selected from knowing the patient's prior experience with these NSAID agents. One of the selected anti-inflammatory agents is given once a day. If pain and inflammation has increased, two of the selected NSAID's may be used according to individual need. On better days with fewer symptoms, the patient can use one or none, commensurate with how he feels, and how effective the medication has been in the past. This orderly sequence is strictly counter to how drugs were prescribed in the past. It was originally considered important to build an effective blood level with these drugs to suppress the inflammatory state. This is considered not a truly effective way to use NSAID drugs. It is more likely that, in time, the individual's disease will develop resistance, or the drug will lose its effectiveness. With prolonged use, many often develop gastropathy with major GI problems.

A next major decision is to decide which drug to begin administering in order to suppress, alter, and potentially quiet the disease. In the past, the list was Plaquenil, Azulfidine, Gold, Cytoxan, or Imuran. All these not only are minimally effective, they and are ever so slow in becoming effective, so the selection has now changed and broadened, Methotrexate had been the agent of choice for nearly twenty five years: this is changing. Broadening is taking place with the use of modern agents that are far superior to any suppressive agents ever employed before. The first of these modern anti-rheumatic drugs generally utilized was Arava; it was then followed with Enbrel, Humira, or Remicade. This represents a large package of anti-disease agents to be programmed into the patient. Far from it a therapeutic program that is customized to the individual and the character of the disease presently represents once being an untreatable disease Rheumatoid Arthritis.

However, over this same period, it has been shown that the more people utilizing the drug, and the longer individuals were on Methotrexate, the more failures were seen. Some patients did not respond and others on the drug for long periods began to lessen the satisfactory response they originally had.

It was at this time, that three successfully designed and clinically effective anti-TNF-α agents were specifically marketed for the treatment of Rheumatoid Arthritis. The administration of these drugs is still relatively early; yet there is a great deal to learn about these biological drugs. The first adverse effect limiting utilization is the cumulative development of allergic reactions, a critical management problem. With their very positive effects in treating arthritis generally, these allergies necessitated either altering the drug, or handing it a stop signal. The alternative selected was correlated to the magnitude of the allergy and its persistence, or degree.

The three innovative drugs, Enbrel, Humira, and Remicade, have totally altered how Rheumatoid Arthritis is to be managed. These drugs are in their infancy regarding their efficacy and long-term outcomes. Not only do we not know the result but also, we still have not established their best therapeutic doses. Every anti-TNF-α agent has its standard manufacturer's dose, and its given frequency for administration to manage Rheumatoid Arthritis. Already, to the consternation of the pay agents, and to the surprise of the manufacturer, the prescribed doses are not accurate. This comes as no surprise to practitioners since all drugs and doses must be related to both patient severity, and disease specificity. More clinical study is needed to reveal the true value of these agents and their long-term resultants.

As mentioned and illustrated, recommended prescribed doses seldom if ever correspond to Rheumatologic reality. The disease is so uniquely individual, that only time will dictate how much and in what combinations of multiple drugs will be effective. As soon as these new disease-modifying agents arrived, we discover responses were wide and varied!

The previously mentioned is well illustrated by the Kineret story. One of the most interesting areas of wonderment was the roll of Kineret, an interleukin-1 receptor antagonist. From the data of all early biochemical and immunological research investigations, Kineret should have been the perfect agent to treat Inflammatory Arthritis. If this were the case, then why, if it blocks interleukin-1, was its alteration of the disease negligible, if at all? The molecular immunology suggests this should not be so. This clinically illustrates more activity occurs than is presently understood. This further illustrates that even with the exceptional knowledge that is known; immunologically and biologically more knowledge is needed clinically in reference to these drugs.

Because of all the agents and past combinations of them, one wonders if an Interleukin-1 receptor antagonist combined with other agents - even Thalidomide - anti-TNF-α, Arava, or any other substance can work to further inhibit the inflammatory process. One can only speculate how at the molecular level these biochemical substances will effectuate a response in Rheumatoid Arthritis patients.

Combinations being just one speculative area, dosage is another one demanding our consideration. Its clinically obvious already that the dose recommended for the monoclonal antibody that binds TNF-α is not predictable. Combinations in the form of Methotrexate with the standard dose of Remicade are already being utilized effectively. The major question that arises is whether it is more efficacious to raise the dose at its mandated interval, or to maintain that dose at a shorter interval?

Cogent arguments exist for either decision. One might reason: why administer more of a successful drug just hoping it'll last longer when one doesn't know how long it is effective, or what its metabolic result will be? This generates many not easily answered questions.

If the prescribed dose is successful, why not maintain that dose rather than challenge the individual to one with a larger dose risking over dosage and any number of considered consequences. Will this treatment stimulate a further need for binding to TNF-α with more anti-TNF-α creation or will resistance occur? What's the breakdown rate of these anti-TNF-α agents

Considerations such as this are legion. These questions caused one to think about adding combinations to the recommended treatment programs, and to searching out for greater knowledge concerning their therapeutic effects.

There surely are numerous agents waiting to come out of the same sphere from which these molecular biochemical drugs originated. This amplifies our present need to further determine the molecular and biological effect for each of these substances while patients are undergoing treatment – such as where is the medicine or how much is left? Measurements of metabolites are one example of a mechanism to determine how much effective agent remains after administering it, enhancing the ease of dispensation.

Rheumatologists are aware of the fact that anti-TNF-α agents are enhanced when used with Methotrexate. A recent study illustrated that low doses of Methotrexate - in patients with active Rheumatoid Arthritis - decreases the immune activity of T-cell modulators in the active tissue area. At the same time, doses of Methotrexate - in normal individuals - stimulates the immune system to react. These contra-indicative data suggest it acts as a foreign agent. This possibly explains why large doses of Methotrexate aren't necessary, and are probably responsible for the side-effects that sometimes result. This adds to understanding why, when Methotrexate is added to anti-TNF-α agents, the dampening of T-cell activity occurs along with the blocking of TNF-α: it's attacking the disease at its origin, and where it causes damage. Does this represent an early rudimentary learning of the mechanism of treating the bimolecular immunological cause of Rheumatoid Arthritis?

These new agents combined with the older agents are the most effective drugs that have arrived on the Rheumatoid Arthritis' management scene. Our field has been energized, but we need more than the drugs: we need working prescriptions. This requires freedom to use the agents in a variety of doses, and in a variety of combinations. We then will know, to a useful degree, the safety, and effect of the treatment. Manufacturers face the task of providing an environment that makes these drugs more readily available to those who are in need. A solution to very expensive administering cost may lie in altering doses and fostering combinations of proven lower priced drugs. Such programs offer a grand possibility that cost can be contained. And with lower cost, great use generating lower costs and expanded applicability.

The anti-TNF-α drugs are the closest we've come to answering what is the mechanics of the specific causative agents bringing damage to inflamed joints. Now what is desperately needed is increased ease of administration with increased numbers of patients on these drugs.

Active treatment results in learning more about the effectiveness of dosages. Added to that is the variability of all patients with Rheumatoid Arthritis. Already it appears that all the specific agents, such as Enbrel, Remicade, and Humira, will have made advances far beyond one's original imagination. Just as it appears cause and answers are near, with knowledge of T-cell activity known, the question of the immune systems B-cell, and the why of their antibodies, enters the picture.

When the mantel of fear of litigation is lifted, greater information about these important drugs will be known, and added to management.

CHAPTER 13
BIOLOGICAL MANAGEMENT and OUR FUTURE TREATMENT of AUTOIMMUNE IMMUNOLOGIC DISEASES

Before embarking into this chapter's major theme, Immunologic drugs, it seems important to recount elements of Immunogenetic disease. These diseases and the havoc perpetuated on many a patient by treating them have taught us a great deal. Lessons taught us in getting to Rheumatoid Arthritis' present state will demonstrate how far we had come even before this era of biologic drugs came to be.

Modern Rheumatology has had some medical misdirection's.

- Cortisone was hailed as a cure until extended use severely affected its patients' bodies.
- One of the earliest procedures that were no less mutilating was the full mouth extraction. During the period, when oral hygiene was not yet in vogue, removal of a focus of infection was tried in those with Rheumatoid Arthritis. There was always an attempt to ascertain a cause, and an infected mouth focused a suspicion that it was possibly a cause of stimulating or enhancing the disease.
- The specific antigen that causes Inflammatory Arthritis has been considered an infection since the result looks and acts as an infectious process.
- Chemicals viruses and a combination of the mentioned have been thought of and as those mentioned however none have been documented.
- There is definite suggestive evidence that there is some familial tendency in these immunological autoimmune diseases and Inflammatory Arthritis. It has been described that in monozygotic twins (twins from a single ovum) that, if one has Inflammatory Arthritis (RA), the other has a 25% chance of developing RA.

It is declared the genetic risk for RA is found in the particular alleles (forms of a gene occupying the same position on paired chromosomes and controlling a characteristic) of the class III major history-compatibility complex (MCH).

A BIT OF ELEMENTARY BACKGROUND DATA ABOUT OUR IMMUNE SYSTEM

Long extensive research has defined many of the effects of immune cells as monocytes, macrophages, T-cells and B-cells formed to destroy antigens but sometimes a good cell, like in synovial tissues, gets permanently defined as an antigen to be eliminated. The complex products of these secretory proinflammatory cytokines, such as IL-1, IL-6, IL-8, IL-10, and TNF-α, are the product of the inflammatory process.

Many attempts have been made to determine what stimulates or enhances this inflammatory progression. As yet we have not been able to ascertain why these autoantibodies are produced, and are so destructive.

Recent specific countering of autoantibodies represents a unique stage in this area of medicine. Our particular autoimmune disease had originally been defined and categorically labeled by its end-stage result. Rheumatoid Arthritis became characteristically synonymous with severely deformed joints. This disability and disfiguring event was the end damage not the symptomatic onset of arthritic joints. The mechanism of synovial inflammation and the damage that occurs to the joint structures is, we further understand, a molecular result of inflammation. It's because of this that, earlier in this manuscript, we defined a more descriptive and clinical categorization of this disease as an autoimmune Immunogenetic disease with various stages and classification rather than continuing to use the term: Rheumatoid Arthritis [except to ease speech].

This broader insight into and knowledge of autoimmune diseases provides us with a different thought about these diseases. The immune system and the knowledge regarding the complicated biological and intricate immunologic effect of the act of inflammation demonstrate these events and how individualistic are these entities. Each incident of inflammatory disease is an individual expression of that disease, making each assessment just as unique. Every one with these diseases finds it being expressed differently.

This concept offers greater credence to the fact that these diseases must be managed individually so that management needs to be customized to the individual. The problem arises about how to use drugs with prescribed doses. As our industry is developing new biological drugs to treat inflammatory disease an emerging conflict between mandated and clinically devised patient prescriptions is emerging evermore obviously. These drugs each have FDA approval for a specific disease. They do not have labeled approval for other related autoimmune inflammatory conditions. Three drugs: Enbrel, Remicade, and Humira are specific for cytokine molecular blocking in explicit diseases using specified doses. These drugs block TNF-α that causes joint and cartilage damage.

But their drug labels add great specificity to treating Inflammatory Arthritis even though not each condition has the same actual degree of inflammation, and the amount of TNF-α precisely occurring in each event is different. The dose of anti-TNF-α needed for each such arthritic event is individually expressed in each patient. One must think of each autoimmune disease afflicted patient as an individual. This runs counter to the present-day labeling of a standard dose for a categorized diagnosis as if dosing was one for all, and all for one.

After years of treatment and management of autoimmune and inflammatory diseases, it's become clear that off-label use of drugs in treatment was the norm. It's also known that as dramatic and unique as the new biological drugs are, their response is not as complete as originally contrived. With the exceptional diagramming and mapping of the specific molecular blocking, it might be assumed, these diseases are now beautifully controlled. The Kineret story described earlier offers a worrisome analogy that total control may not be the case for all the agents.

Further experience has illustrated the labeled dose is only modestly unique. For example, Enbrel can be effective at half the suggested dose, and can even be taken at wider intervals for a mild disease. On the other hand at its full-recommended dose, it can be both effective and full of side effects. Humira has similar characteristics: to control the inflammatory process, half and double doses are more often needed than is recorded. Remicade remains the single one of the newer biological drugs that can have ease of titrating the dose to the patients need. This resulted from years of persuasively counseling third parties, such as the manufacturer and insurance companies to comply with their need.

Another interesting anecdote in reference to these new biological drugs is that experience with long-term use illustrates fluid retention. This can occur in many areas and the most common is the lower extremity. Other tissues noted have been the perineum, and even generalized with seeming unexplained weight gain. This could be part of the explanation of CNS (Central nervous system) problems and headache, which is quite common. Many times after these undesired effects occur patients can still tolerated the drug with almost half the original dose. Even more enlightening is the lesser dose seems to maintain its effectiveness. These findings are not highlighted by the manufacturer, which again illustrates the value of clinical assessment and the illogic of standardized treatment. Beyond that the question of tolerance and accommodations to the drug long-term use seems to definitely change. One cannot help but punctuate the fact that standard doses are fallacious in fact and recent government and Medicare attacks at off label use and limitations is counter to good clinical management.

ARTHROCENTESIS AND JOINT INJECTION

There now are more definitive and specific uses of the biological drugs. They should be supplied in multiple doses so as to have the best-determined individual use, and to allow for alternate routes of administration. Providing smaller and larger doses makes them available for milder disease, and for those requiring larger dosage. The intent, as has frequently been mentioned, is to protect the joint and the cartilage from minimal but progressive damage. What is being suggested is to consider utilizing an off-label area for these agents.

With that in mind let's hearken back to Arthritis' cortisone experience. After originally feeling that the cure had finally come, nothing but problems began surfacing from prolonged high doses use, and the disease was no longer being curtailed. Cortisone demonstrated the greatest anti-inflammatory effect and nothing has approached cortisone in that regard since. Years of experience with cortisone had shown that small doses of crystalline cortisone instilled directly into the joint had dramatic anti-inflammatory effects. This had and has widespread effect but this good news could not tunnel through the banter regarding its use because of is early serious problem. For many years this has been a cornerstone of Rheumatology's treating of severe swelling and synovitis in isolated joints. Although this treatment is very effective symptomatically it has no known definitive effect on truly altering the disease process within the joint.

Extrapolating this experience of placing therapeutic agents directly into the joint opens the mind to formulating other ways of using these new biological drugs. As more fully explained earlier, they act directly on the synovial tissue by attacking the inflammatory event that lies behind Inflammatory Arthritis. An awareness of the unique molecular blockage that protects against the ultimate cartilage and joint damage creates a thought. Why not place a small amount of this effective agent directly into the joint so as to act directly where its effect is desired?

This leads to considering how and what could be used to instill into a joint that would locally produce the desired effect, but are now used by injecting that agent parentally as a subcutaneous infusion. Each of the four biological drugs was considered.

- When injected, Kineret is very painful and on adding in the experience that it doesn't provide a clinically positive effect it was immediately discounted.
- Remicade is intravenously injected but small doses are not available. With further consideration however it is not harmful given IV. If it were ever available in such a form it may be the best drug to be used in the way just contemplated.

- Humira is long acting and has a preservative and not in an aqueous solution. This is not an entirely negative reason for not using it but it requires deeper consideration.
- Finally, Enbrel is the most logical of the biological drugs to consider for this means of administration. It's soluble in water, and dosing is not difficult. Originally, it was distributed as a crystalline substance to be dissolved in sterile water producing 1cc of Enbrel (equivalent to 25 mgm). This is the state of the medication injected subcutaneously.

The initial consideration was to:

- Ascertain if the agent was painful, or irritating to the joint,
- If there was any after effect,
- What positive effect was produced, if any?

The next step was finding an isolated joint that had an easily perceived synovitis. As frequently noted, to test the use of intra-articular agent [like Enbrel] on a synovial joint, a knee was the most logical selection. A knee, which is swollen and has palpable synovitis is tender, limited in range of motion, and has easily felt warmth. In addition, the subject will notice aching while resting in bed at night. The slightest motion brings pain with a general aching in the knee. In order to test how a small dose of Enbrel will be effective in a swollen joint with synovitis a subject must be carefully selected.

The third step was to find a patient[18.] who has had Enbrel and for some reason the route and dose was not the most efficient. The selected subject had the symptoms described, and only one joint was involved. Subcutaneous Enbrel was parentally given at 12.5 mgm with a definite clinical response. The symptoms in fact diminished by about 80%. Swelling, aching, pain, and joint function all improved. This was used on demand with the dose being adjusted according to the symptoms, and at a need-determined interval. Shortly after the dose sinus congestion occurred which was originally considered the beginning of a sinus infection. Within a day it subsided and was discounted until it was repeated following each Enbrel injection. This specific reaction is one of the common side effects infrequently noted by the manufacturer.

Because the Enbrel was effective - when given sub-q in small intermittent doses for the isolated synovitis – an analogous alternative was considered: a small dose of Humira was tried. This was as effective as the

---

[18.] With confidence, desire to learn about the procedure and a direct need the author was the fist patient to encounter this procedure. This was the first subject to have intermittent injected small doses of Enbrel for a degenerative joint disease of the knee with associated synovitis.

Enbrel and used intermittently in a small dose. After a few injections, the subject developed a slight bronchial congestion for a day or so. This also was a known allergic effect of Humira. It was so clinically effective; the subject was not pleased there was no other alternative to treat the synovitis. This was directed locally at a moderately degenerated knee joint with the specific treatment as needed. The rationale behind the use of the drug in this fashion wasn't only to control the symptoms, but a mechanism of shrinking the synovitis thereby protecting the articular cartilage against further damage from wear and tear [a clinical term for use and abuse] thereby preventing an ultimate joint replacement.

The first time this was preformed 10 mgm of Enbrel was injected into the knee after a small amount of synovial fluid was removed. As expected, the result was as effective. The synovitis was markedly diminished as were the symptoms described: heat, swelling, night aching pain, soreness and stiffness. The pattern that followed was: Enbrel being given in doses of 5 to 10 mgm according to the quality and quantity of synovitis clinically detected. Over the last 24 to 36 months, this has been done approximately every month or two according to clinical need with doses determined by the clinical state.

Since then, at least 200 patients have had over 380 joint injections of Enbrel with the just-stated doses. A more complete clinical description of all the injections will be tabulated in a later publication. There were no side effects in these treated patients as their synovitis decreased. In some instances, it was as effective as a steroid injection. Infused Enbrel's finest potential effect lies in cartilage protection. It's alleged that synovitis weakens the cartilage, predisposing it to further damage. That being the case, this manner of using Enbrel could be the easiest and one of the more effective ways of employing Enbrel for isolated-joint synovitis. If maintaining the integrity of articular cartilage is paramount, it matters little if the underlying problem is Inflammatory Arthritis or Degenerative Joint Disease (DJD). It has been used in both early and late DJD. The conclusion was that it unquestionably reduced the synovitis physically, and clinically. The key is educating all to think in terms of joints clinically with synovitis and not in terms of arthritic names.

As a follow-up, a small number of patients have had 10 mgm of Humira injected into the knee or ankle. This produced a similar clinical effect. Some of the subjects had a satisfactory effect while some claimed no effective response. One of the problems in evaluation the result is having the patient differentiate the pain from synovitis compared to the mechanical pain effect present in arthritis. Quite importantly: no side effects have been detected.

With this reasonable clinical observation, couldn't it be reasonably assume that Enbrel's manufacturer, in some way or other, would respond to this experience? In fact the company was not only disinterested, they refused to discuss these data. It even refused to hear of the special way the drug was being used and its effectiveness. This may sound bizarre, but one must take into consideration they are not interested in new and unique uses of the drug, even if sales and profits increase. Drug companies fear the so-called off-label use of drugs. Their fears arise from finding problems that cause a loss of FDA approval, and loss of the drug itself. Unhappily, this seemingly wild, unwarranted fear has previously been awarded its warrants.

Vioxx provides a recent example of our loss of a great anti-inflammatory drug. Fear of class action lawsuits from armies of litigators dumped this promising arthritic pain reliever into the refuse burring valley once called Gehenna. Enbrel's - and other biological agents' - additional potential effective, safe uses in joints, do need further clinical support by pharmaceutical companies. But because of out present litigious environment, it may not see full evaluation for years.

All these new biological drugs with their known modes of action could be used in any number of other inflamed areas. Under the present climate of litigation fear, it may take a long time before these exciting agents are used to there fullest, and in varied doses, or even for Immunogenetic ailments. These biological drugs are of great interest with a new management and treatment avenue by blocking specific molecular agents that cause tissue damage. This is now taking treatment directly into the diseased tissue, and identifying how tissue damage occurs and the result of that damage.

This is a new horizon in medicine and the arthritic patient is the first recipient of this new era in medicine.

MYOSITIS

Advances in modern medicine come to pass through thought, courage, and trial-and-error.

Another area where the new anti-TNF-α blocking drugs were used is in the constellation of myositis diseases. This term arises from its end-stage inclusions in the muscle. Specifically, IBM or Inclusion Body Myositis is a muscle disease that is promoted as one where the muscle is damaged by the mysterious inclusion of material into the muscle cell, resulting in weakness and permanent muscle damage. This is diagnosed by muscle biopsy.

Two patients who carried this diagnosis were originally seen. The majority of symptoms were lower extremity weakness, loss of power and strength in hand and upper extremity, smooth muscle problems with swallowing. Further evaluation revealed the disease was also diagnosed using muscle biopsy. Incidentally, there were elevated CPK (phosphocreatine kinase) values. Both patients were under the care of neurologists, and were told there is not a know treatment for IBM. This constellation of symptoms, findings, and laboratory tests illustrate much of the problem of management and treatment of autoimmune diseases.

This seemed incredible no-treatment diagnostic or even clinically tried agents were suggested. There was an implication that something was amiss with this problematic disease. Polymyositis was and is a relatively known entity in rheumatology. Consequently, Rheumatologists evaluated these two cases. The biopsy was reviewed, the patients were examined, and laboratory tests were review. The study so-gathered pronounced that the most startling event was profound muscle weakness and its progression. This was associated with high CPK enzymes. Review of the muscle biopsy report revealed that inflammatory cells present in the muscles with inclusion bodies were present.

The supposition was **what if** this IBM disease was not a specific inclusion body disease whereby, for some metabolic reason yet unexplained, an amyloidal substance is deposited in muscle causing it's death. Such analysis is the consequence of looking at the end result of damaged muscle with inclusion bodies, but that actually followed muscle inflammation with muscle damage suggested by the elevated CPK. It was supposed this was an example of labeling the disease by the end result. In essence it is polymyositis: inflamed damaged muscles often already diseased with inclusion bodies at the end of the process. This suggests that this is an autoimmune disease; therefore the inflammatory cells here were releasing cytokines just as are Inflammatory Arthritis cells. That being the case, should not this disease also respond to immunosuppression, and cytokine blocking?

Here these cases were diagnostically labeled by an end-result. From the findings, they could be amenable to immunosuppressive and biological drugs to treat this condition off-label. Please recall our earlier discussion concerning handing end-stage names to disease, as in the early diagnosis of Rheumatoid Arthritis. Left out of that preceding discussion was an unnamed state of Inflammatory Arthritis. This is what arthritis was before its name evolves into RA.

Having received this correlation and, following discussion and education with patients and physicians, treatment began with a standard biweekly 25 mgm dose of Enbrel with a weekly 7.5 mgm dose of Methotrexate. After four to six months, a dramatic improvement of skeletal and smooth muscle weakness, which had previously been dramatically disabling, and strength and swallowing improved. In time, there was very remarkable improvement of skeletal muscle weakness in walking and hand function.

As their improvement progressed, with clinical gains in strength, the CPK fell dramatically. These unexpected clinical advances quickly spread their information through the associations of inflicted patients. Interest strongly developed about the thought process provoking this alternative, resulting in other people being evaluated. A starting dose these agent were custom designed to fit each individual case. Muscle biopsies of all patients were positive just like the patients originally treated. The therapy has been considered a clinical trial of Methotrexate and a biological agent to determine if suppression of the suspected polymyositis will respond. All its sufferers are eagerly waiting to see the results of this clinical trial, as are others having an autoimmune disease. This experience is promoting clinical thinking in many areas.

- Our still archaic method of naming diseases needs to be changed as in diagnosing Inflammatory Synovitis as RA.
- IBM may not be a unique disease, but a state of muscle Polymyositis. (*Only the author has suggested this and it is challenged by the IBM organization and others*)
- Off-label use of drugs should be given greater consideration in situations that have the essence of clinical indications.
- The final chapter on these presented concepts on arthritis and other unique cases is waiting to be written.

CONCLUDING REMARKS

Medical reporting of data that doesn't fit tradition finds extreme difficulty in gaining recognition. All the modern ideas, and treatments presented in this monograph are attempts to present new concepts and terminology. A presentation of clinically proven information to our leading figures of authority has been denied or ignored. That will change. While leaving these anecdotal mentioned events with myositis, is worth brief mention similar experiences have been noted with diseases as Scleroderma and Lupus Erythematosus (again end stage names and terms).

Investigations such as clinical trials or off-label use of drugs are looked upon askance. The traditional investigations of drugs that are given greatest credibility are the so-called double blind studies. Drug companies are extremely sensitive about how drugs trials are to be done. Their constraints preclude off-label trials because by its off-label title alone, they may be used in treating diseases for which that drug had not been tested and so lacks approval. (Devil's Claw, because it has no FDA label, can be sold to treat any disease, and is).

Laying behind on-labels constraints is a good protective thing a customary FDA requirement: double-blind testing of any drug sold or used on the open market. Such studies for off-label use only result after a drug has been in use for many years. In our day and age, especially with regard to new biological drugs, these agents do not seem to stand a chance for being considered for off-label use. The biological drugs being so specifically designed to pick a definitive molecule to block in a known disease are everywhere on-label. In addition, the biological drugs are expensive and third party payers will always reject unlabelled treatment. Only the manufacturer could perform or permit such a study. Have we here a double negative further hindering clinical trials?

The future is just at the start of this era of biological agents that will be affecting the immune system to control many of the multiple autoimmune diseases with these drugs. Coming forth are many other and likely even more novel and more specific newer biological drugs.

Orencia (abatacept) is another infusion drug. The manufacturer labels it as the first in a class that differs from any other agent used for Inflammatory Arthritis (RA). The manufacturer states that this agent targets the co-stimulation of T-cells. This occurs further *upstream* in the inflammatory state, and helps effect the *downstream* Interleukins where the cytokines are, i.e. TNF-α and other multiple effects of inflammation.

One descriptive of this and other such drugs - when using the term downstream - follows. As the inflammatory cells act and react in response to an antigen's stimulus, numerous biochemical, and cellular, effects and reactions occur. T-cells from the Thymus Gland and B-cells from the Bone Marrow become involved in protecting the body against foreign prowlers. They produce cytokines one of which TNF-α is the resulting molecule. These are the substances that are being blocked by the biological agents that were the main subject of these last two chapters. Further back in the inflammatory reaction are the upstream cells mentioned earlier so their anti-inflammatory effect is less specific.

Rituxan (rituximab) is another recently released agent. It's also an infusion drug; it depletes B-cells, and is also used to treat non-Hodgkin's lymphoma. It's administered in two infusions according to weight and is claimed to have lasting effects.

Two others [yet to be released] agents are Certolizumab (Cimzia), a monthly injection that also blocks TNF-α.

The other new drug specifically acts to block another cytokine Interleukin-6. These various cytokine blockers being studied strengthen the perceived problems clinicians face while further demonstrating the complexity of the inflammation process, the individuality of the autoimmune diseases, and showing a tip of our iceberg waiting to float ashore.

The thesis of the manuscript have been attempting to present the future of Rheumatology and its allied disciplines, as well as to illustrate how there is great potential for treatment and management of the autoimmune inflammatory disease. Today, however, many are diagnostically saddled over a burr that labels end-stage diagnoses as the diseases. Many of these basic immunologic diseases could be helped, if the biological drugs used in trial-tests of a variety of customized doses. The reason for making an issue of off-label uses with variable doses is because for each individual patient, his particular disease expresses itself individually. In accepting this, treatment and the drugs can be individually tried using clinically designed customized doses.

By using mandated doses, some can be over medicated and suffer side effects like allergic reactions. Such effects many halt its personal use so that its therapeutic effect is denied. Before these agents are tried on the unique autoimmune disease, a double blind study should be done. These are drugs that have already been released by the FDA, but now need clinical usage and clinical trials.

Another case that exemplifies one of modern medicine's cul-de-sacs discussed earlier is the fad diagnosis Polymyalgia Rheumatica (PMR). Its patients have joint symptoms that are modest in nature. They are patients with muscle aching and weakness symptoms. Laboratory test usually show a very high sedimentation rate. When this was first written of in the literature as a new disease, its only suggested treatment was large doses of steroids. It was considered this was the way to manage the disease just like in the 1950's when Cortisone was given for Inflammatory Arthritis (RA). That treatment was handed the Nobel Prize for Medicine before its failure was apparent. That suggested treatment of PMR with cortisone just covers it as had been detailed within this manuscript.

When carefully examined, many PMR patients with these symptoms will demonstrate mild swelling and perceptible synovitis. There can also be a mild elevation of the CPK, which demonstrates they have an Inflammatory Synovitis and Myositis. Rather than a vague non-anatomical descriptive label as its name, one more descriptive of what is physically occurring is called for. If one cares to combine the two expressions of the autoimmune disease, Mixed Inflammatory Tissue Disease is clearer.

There are many non-conventional thoughts and ideas all of which are complimented by about forty years of clinical experience. We end with the beginning statement about opinion written by John Stuart Mill.

> *"The peculiar evil of silencing the expression of an opinion is, that it is robbing the human race; posterity as well as the existing generation; those who dissent from the opinion, still more than those who hold it. If the opinion is right, they are deprived of the opportunity of exchanging error for truth, if wrong, they lose, what is almost as great a benefit, the clearer perception and livelier impression of truth, produced by its collision with error".*

GLOSSARY

HEALTH ORGANIZATIONS
AASCRD *American Association for the Study and Control of Rheumatic Diseases*
ACR   *American College of Rheumatology*
ARE   *American Rheumatism Association*
CDC   *Center for Disease Control & prevention*
FDA   *Federal Drug Administration*
NIH   *National Institute of Health*

DRUG TYPES
Anti-tumor Necrosis Factor alpha *(anti-TNF-α.) – this is the biological antibody produced to block the damaging molecule (TNF-α) in arthritic joints.*
DMARD's, *(disease modifying and remitting drugs)* example agents are Plaquenil, Cupramine, Asulfadine, Cytoxan, Imuran and more.
NSAID's, *Non-Steroidal Anti-Inflammatory Drugs sixteen or more of such Motrin and allied drugs.*
Steroids, *local acting, Aristacort or DepoMedrol;*

ARTHRITIC DISEASES AND NAMES
Acute iridocyclitis *– acute inflammation of the iris and ciliary body of the eye.*
Ankylosing Spondylitis *– arthritis of the spine resulting in rigidity of the spine also called (Rheumatoid Spondylitis; Spondylitis, spondylarthropathy)*
Arthrocentesis *– introduction of a needle into a joint to remove fluid to determine what is occurring in the joint.*
Baker's Cyst accumulation *of fluid behind the knee communicating with the knee joint.*
Bamboo Spine *– fused rigid spine appearing like a bamboo pole on x-ray*
Capelins Syndrome *– condition of large pulmonary nodules in RA patients exposed to coal dust.*
Carpal Tunnel Syndrome *– compression of the median nerve at the wrist under the carpel ligament usually due to inflammation in the wrist.*
Crohn's disease *– chronic inflammation of the terminal small intestine and the large Colon - the large intestine*
Cushing's disease *– disorder caused by excessive cortisone causing moon face and many other abnormal finding due to excessive cortisone effect on the body.*

Diabetes mellitus – *condition of lack of insulin from the pancreatic Islets of Langerhan causing elevated blood sugar*

Epstein-Barr – *virus that causes infection*

Erosive Osteoarthritis – *condition of degenerative changes of the proximal and distal small joints of the fingers with x-ray evidence of erosions.*

Fibromyalgia – *vague term to describe a wide variety of symptoms of the neck muscles and joints that are most likely mild inflammatory arthritis undiagnosed.*

Fibrositis – *older term of a condition of symptoms similar to the above*

Ganglion – *cyst on the tendon usually in the wrist.*

Glomerulonephritis – *inflammation of the area of the kidney called the glomerulus, which is made of small vessels.*

Gout – *a form of arthritis cause by elevated uric acid depositing in the joint.*

Guillain-Barré, - *a peripheral neuritis spreading to the trunk called ascending paralysis, which is of unknown cause and frequently fully reversible.*

Hypertrophic Osteoarthritis - *DJD, which is arthritis, associated with cartilage degeneration.*

Hyperuricemia *(high uric acid)*

IBM – *(Inclusion Body Myositis)*

Inflammatory Arthritis *hypersensitivity inflammatory state of the synovial joints and specific name for mild Rheumatoid Arthritis*

Juvenile Rheumatoid Arthritis *JRA or juvenile chronic polyarthritis, and Still's disease*

Kidney stones, *renal calculi that can be due to calcium and or uric acid*

Lateral epicondylitis *inflammation of the outside of the elbow.*

Lupus Erythematosus; *SLE; drug-induced lupus erythematosus;*

Mixed Connective Tissue Disease – *inflammation condition, which has characteristic of RA, Lupus, and the other connective diseases, which cannot be separated clinically.*

Multiple sclerosis, - *progressive disease of the nervous system involving the brain an Nerves causing many diagnostic clinical and MRI changes.*

Myositis – *An autoimmune disease with generalized muscle weakness and unlimited permanent muscle damage.*

Neuropathic arthritis – *arthritis attributed to joint damage because of severe neuritis associated with diabetes and characterized by damage appearing beyond just trauma.*

Olecranon bursitis a *fluid collection in the bursa at the elbow. Usually from trauma*

Osteoarthritis – *arthritis from cartilage degeneration*

<u>Osteomyelitis</u> – *infection of the bone*

<u>Osteoporosis</u> – *a condition of demineralization of the bone usually after menopause and can be caused by cortisone excess.*

<u>Paget's disease</u> – a *disease of bone causing deformity and disorganized bone structure.*

<u>Podagra</u> – *attack of acute gouty arthritis of the great toe of the joint.*

<u>Polymyalgia Rheumatica</u> - *a descriptive name for form of inflammatory arthritis or RA*

<u>Psoriatic Arthritis</u> – *a form of arthritis with psoriasis and distinctive joint changes.*

<u>Reiter's syndrome</u> – *a form of arthritis associated with a constellation of symptoms and bowel symptoms and mucous membrane involvement*

<u>Reye's Syndrome</u> *severe systemic condition in children multisystem and less common now and attributed to a virus and post aspirin use.*

<u>Rheumatoid and inflammatory arthritis</u> – *inflammation of joint synovial tissue*

<u>Rheumatoid Arthritis</u> – *destructive inflammatory joint disease.*

<u>Scleroderma</u> - (*Systemic sclerosis (Scleroderma), CREST syndrome, Progressive Systemic Sclerosis) – inflammation of the skin as an autoimmune disease causing scaring of the skin and other systemic findings.*

<u>Ulnar nerve entrapment</u> – *entrapment of the ulnar nerve at the elbow causing numbness of the fourth and fifth fingers of the hand.*

SUBJECT INDEX